TOPICS IN
CLINICAL UROLOGY

EVALUATION AND TREATMENT OF URINARY INCONTINENCE

TOPICS IN CLINICAL UROLOGY

Series Editors
Martin I. Resnick, M.D.
Jack S. Elder, M.D.

New Techniques in Reconstructive Urology
Jack W. McAninch, M.D.

Complications of Interventional Techniques
Culley C. Carson III, M.D.

Pediatric Urology for the General Urologist
Jack S. Elder, M.D.

New Diagnostic Tests
Martin I. Resnick, M.D.
J. Patrick Spirnak, M.D.

New Developments in the Management of Urolithiasis
James E. Lingeman, M.D.
Glenn M. Preminger, M.D.

Medical and Surgical Management of Prostate Cancer
Richard G. Middleton, M.D.

Techniques for Ablation of Benign and Malignant Prostate Tissue
Joseph A. Smith, Jr., M.D.
Douglas F. Milam, M.D.

Evaluation and Treatment of Urinary Incontinence
Jerry G. Blaivas, M.D.

TOPICS IN
CLINICAL UROLOGY

EVALUATION AND TREATMENT OF URINARY INCONTINENCE

Jerry G. Blaivas, M.D., F.A.C.S.

Clinical Professor of Urology
Cornell University Medical School
Attending Urologist
The New York Hospital/Cornell Medical Center
New York, New York

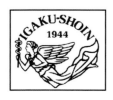

IGAKU-SHOIN   NEW YORK • TOKYO

Published and distributed by

IGAKU-SHOIN Medical Publishers, Inc.
One Madison Avenue, New York, New York 10010

IGAKU-SHOIN Ltd.,
5-24-3 Hongo, Bunkyo-ku, Tokyo 113–91.

Library of Congress Cataloging-in-Publication Data

Evaluation and treatment of urinary incontinence / [edited by] Jerry
   G. Blaivas.
      p.   cm. — (Topics in clinical urology)
   Includes bibliographical references and index.
   1. Urinary incontinence.   I. Blaivas, Jerry G.   II. Series.
   [DNLM: 1. Urinary Incontinence—therapy.   2. Urinary Incontinence—
diagnosis.   WJ 146 E92 1996]
   RC921.I5E93   1996
   616.6′2—dc20
   DNLM/DLC   96-4750
   for Library of Congress   CIP

ISBN: 0-89640-306-8   (New York)
ISBN: 4-260-14306-9   (Tokyo)

Printed and bound in the U.S.A.
10 9 8 7 6 5 4 3 2 1

PREFACE

No one dies of urinary incontinence. It does not cause cancer; it does not cause pain. At least not the kind of pain that requires narcotics or nonsteroidal anti-inflammatory agents. But it causes pain of another kind, one that leads to embarrassment, psychosocial maladjustment, and isolation. Incontinence afflicts up to 5% of males before the fifth decade of life and about 25% of females in the same age group. Over the age of 60 about 15% of males are afflicted and in females the rate is more than twice that. Incontinence remains the most common reason for institutionalization of the elderly.

To the scientist, these are afflicted males and females; to the physician, the nurse, and other health care professionals, but most of all, to their families, they are actually people. They are girls and boys, men and women, mothers, fathers; and grandparents who, in the more severe cases, tread quiet lives of self-conscious awareness. They plan their days around the availability of bathrooms, packing shopping bags and suitcases full of pads, appliances, and undergarments, but all too often, they just stay home.

Surveys of physicians consistently demonstrate that only about 2% of urologists and 1% of gynecologists in the United States profess a major interest in the diagnosis and treatment of urinary incontinence. Apparently, it is a bit too mundane, too basic. After all, no one dies of urinary incontinence and it does not cause cancer.

This book has three goals, to educate, to educate, and to educate. The first goal is to educate the general reader that caring for patients with incontinence is a most intellectually challenging and psychologically gratifying endeavor. The second goal is to educate the clinician that urinary incontinence is eminently diagnosable in a most straightforward and logical way. The third goal is to educate both the general and more sophisticated reader that urinary incontinence is eminently treatable provided that two ingredients are present—a knowledgeable and motivated clinician and a motivated patient. The congruence of these factors allows each patient to be effectively treated to his or her own level of expectation. Cure is possible in the vast majority of patients, but for many this requires surgery, and many patients choose not to go that route. Nevertheless, with the advent of more effective behavioral and rehabilitative techniques, pharmacologic agents, prosthetic devices, and even better pads and appliances, it is now possible for nearly all patients to be dry.

Jerry G. Blaivas, M.D.

To my coauthors:
My teachers and my friends. The best way to learn is to teach.

CONTRIBUTORS

Rodney A. Appell, M.D., F.A.C.S.
Head, Section of Voiding Dysfunction
    and Female Urology
The Cleveland Clinic Foundation
Cleveland, Ohio

Jerry G. Blaivas, M.D., F.A.C.S.
Clinical Professor of Urology
Cornell University Medical School
Attending Urologist
The New York Hospital/Cornell Medical
    Center
New York, New York

Michael B. Chancellor, M.D.
Associate Professor of Urology
Department of Urology
Jefferson Medical College
Thomas Jefferson University
Philadelphia, Pennsylvania

Ashok Chopra, M.D.
Fellow, Department of Urology
UCLA
University of California for
    Health Sciences
Los Angeles, California

François Haab, M.D.
Urodynamics and Female Urology Fellow
Kaiser Permanente Medical Center
Los Angeles, California

Dianne M. Heritz, M.D., F.R.C.S.C.
Lecturer, University of Toronto
Toronto, Canada

Michael J. Kennelly, M.D.
Division of Urology
The University of Texas–
    Houston Medical School
Houston, Texas

Young Kim, M.D.
Chief Resident, Department of Urology
State University of New York,
    Health Science Center at Brooklyn
Brooklyn, New York

Gary E. Leach, M.D.
Chief, Department of Urology
Kaiser Permanente Medical Center
Clinical Associate Professor of Urology
University of California Los Angeles
Los Angeles, California

Edward J. McGuire, M.D.
Professor and Director
Division of Urology
The University of Texas–
    Houston Medical School
Houston, Texas

Denise A. Nigro, M.D.
Fellow in Urology
University of Pennsylvania Medical
    Center
Philadelphia, Pennsylvania

Victor W. Nitti, M.D.
Assistant Professor, Department of
  Urology
Director of Neurourology and Female
  Urology
New York University Medical Center
New York, New York

Helen E. O'Connell, M.D.
Division of Urology
The University of Texas–
  Houston Medical School
Houston, Texas

Shlomo Raz, M.D.
Professor of Urology
UCLA
University of California
  for Health Sciences
Los Angeles, California

David A. Rivas, M.D.
Assistant Professor of Urology
Department of Urology
Jefferson Medical College
Thomas Jefferson University
Philadelphia, Pennsylvania

Lauri J. Romanzi, M.D., F.A.C.O.G.
Assistant Director, Division of
  Urogynecology
Department of Obstetrics and Gynecology
The New York Hospital/Cornell University
  Medical Center
New York, New York

Diane A. Smith, R.N., M.S.N., C.R.N.P.
Director
Uro Rehab
Bryn Mawr, Pennsylvania

Lynn Stothers, M.D.
Fellow, Department of Urology
UCLA
University of California
  for Health Sciences
Los Angeles, California

Toyohiko Watanabe, M.D., Ph.D.
Neuro-urology and Female Urology
Fellow
Department of Urology
Jefferson Medical College
Thomas Jefferson University
Philadelphia, Pennsylvania

Alan J. Wein, M.D.
Professor and Chair
Division of Urology
University of Pennsylvania Medical
Center
Chief of Urology
Hospital of the University of Pennsylvania
Philadelphia, Pennsylvania

J. Christian Winters, M.D.
Clinical Assistant Professor of Urology
Louisiana State University Medical Center
New Orleans, Louisiana

CONTENTS

EVALUATION AND TREATMENT OF URINARY INCONTINENCE

1

Anatomy and Physiology of the Lower Urinary Tract: Influence on Urinary Continence

Victor W. Nitti
Young Kim

In order to effectively evaluate and treat urinary incontinence, a thorough understanding of the anatomy and physiology of the lower urinary tract is imperative. The basic functions of the lower urinary tract are to store adèquate volumes of urine at low pressure and allow for its voluntary evacuation. Low-pressure storage assures protection of the kidneys and containment of urine within the bladder until voluntary evacuation is desired. Anatomic and functional abnormalities may interfere with the normal delicate balance of storage and emptying and incontinence can result. The causes of incontinence are as numerous as the anatomic and physiologic aberrations that can occur.

The purpose of this chapter will be to summarize the normal anatomy and physiology of the lower urinary tract with respect to urine storage and emptying. Understanding the framework discussed here should assist the reader as specific etiologies and treatments of incontinence are presented later in this text.

Anatomically, with respect to continence, the lower urinary tract can be divided into the bladder and the bladder outlet (bladder neck and urethra). While the anatomy and physiology of the bladder is similar in males and females, the bladder outlet and urethra vary significantly. As a result, while causes of bladder dysfunction are similar among men and women, causes of outlet dysfunction vary greatly. Thus we will begin our discussion with the bladder outlet and continence mechanism in the female, followed by that in the male.

A discussion of the anatomy of pelvic support in the female is included as this is crucial to the maintenance of urinary continence. Finally, we will present the relevant anatomic features of the bladder and a summary of the neurophysiology of normal urinary storage and emptying.

ANATOMY OF THE FEMALE BLADDER OUTLET AND URETHRA

Pelvic Support

More than in the male, the anatomy of the female pelvis is a significant contributor to lower urinary tract function and particularly urinary continence. In females, changes in pelvic support and anatomic relationships occur as a result of childbearing and hormonal changes. The individual organs, their relationship to one another, and their supporting structures are all critical in maintaining continence and normal lower urinary tract function. With respect to urinary continence, the bladder neck and urethra must maintain closure at rest and with increases in abdominal pressure. This will depend on the intrinsic nature of the urethra to maintain a "seal" as well as the integrity of the pelvic floor which must provide support around the bladder neck and proximal urethra and cause it to remain closed during increases in abdominal pressure.

All pelvic structures draw their support from the bony pelvis. Upon this framework, the proximal urethra and bladder are supported by the levator musculature and its various fascial condensations which include the pubourethral ligaments, urethropelvic ligament, pubocervical fascia, and cardinal ligaments. The levator ani muscles provide the principal active inferior support for the urethra, vagina, and rectum. The muscle is divided into three component parts: pubococcygeus, iliococcygeus, and coccygeus (Fig. 1.1). Standard anatomy texts describe the muscle together with its surrounding fascia as a broad thin sheet extending laterally from the pelvic portion of the pubic bone to the symphysis anteriorly, and to the inner surface of the ischial spine posteriorly. Between these points it attaches to another major structural support, the arcus tendineus (Fig. 1.2). This thick fascial band extends between the pubis and ischial spine. Near the pubis, it lies on the inner, medial surface of the levator ani and posteriorly overlies the obturator internus muscle. It is responsible for most of the lateral support. From the tendineus arc the levator fascia, including a component of smooth muscle, extends medially to support the pelvic structures. As it approaches the urethra and bladder it can be thought of as "splitting" to envelop these structures. It becomes the endopelvic fascia on the abdominal side and the fascia of the anterior vaginal wall.

Support of the proximal urethra and bladder neck has been described by Delancey as forming a sling.[1] This sling is attached laterally to the arcus tendineus and is composed of collagen and elastin containing connective tissue and smooth muscle which originates from the detrusor muscle. Delancey refers to this structure as the pubovesical ligament or urethral supports, while Raz calls it the urethropelvic ligament.[2,3,3a,3b] We favor the later term as it has been used extensively in the urologic literature to describe various reconstructive procedures.[4-6] In any event, this structure extends from the proximal and midurethral area and attaches to the arcus tendineus to provide the major support of the bladder neck and proximal urethra (Figs. 1.3 and 1.4). The urethropelvic or vesicopelvic ligament has been shown to be a separate structure from the pubourethral ligaments.[2] The

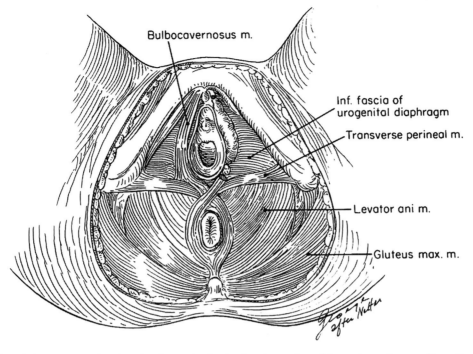

Fig. 1.1. Levator ani and perineal muscles in the female as viewed from the perineum. (From Raz et al, ref. 3, with permission.)

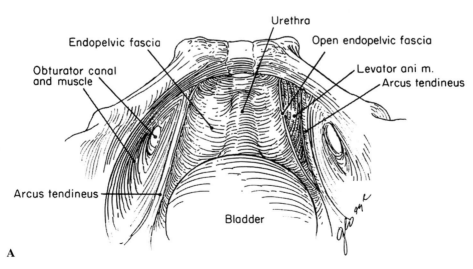

A

Fig. 1.2. A: Retropubic view of levator ani and obturator internus muscles and relationship to arcus tendineus and endopelvic fascia. **B:** Same view with endopelvic fascia removed. (From Raz et al, ref. 3, with permission.)

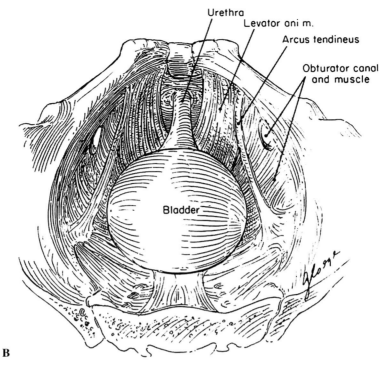

Urethra

Levator ani m.

Arcus tendineus

Obturator canal
and muscle

Bladder

B

Fig. 1.2. B: Continued.

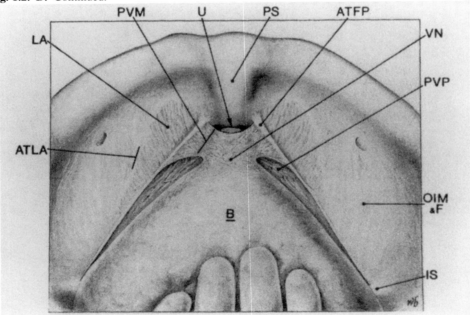

Fig. 1.3. Retropubic view of bladder neck and urethral support drawn from cadaver dissections according to Delancey. The pubovesical muscle (PVM) can be seen going from the vesical neck (VN) to the arcus tendineus fasciae pelvis (ATFP) and running over the paraurethral vascular plexus (PVP). ATLA = arcus tendineus levator ani; B = bladder; IS = ischial spine; LA = levator ani muscle; OIM&F = obturator internus muscle and fascia; PS = pubic symphysis; U = urethra. (From Delancey, ref. 2, with permission.)

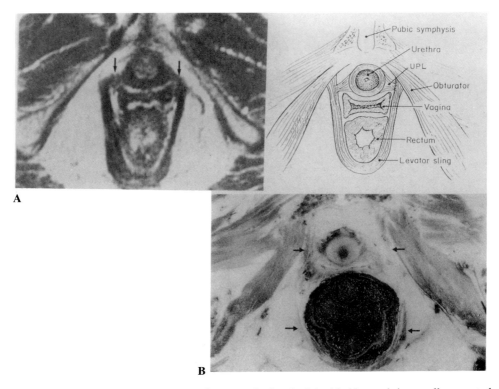

Fig. 1.4. A: Axial magnetic resonance image at the level of the bladder neck in a well-supported continent woman shows urethropelvic ligaments (UPL, *arrows*) supporting bladder neck. **B:** Corresponding step section at same level shows urethropelvic ligaments attaching to the levator (*arrows*) at the level of the arcus tendineus. (From Klutke et al, ref. 3a, with permission.)

posterior pubourethral ligaments are paired bands of dense connective tissue which arise from the vaginal wall and periurethral tissue and are attached to the undersurface of the symphysis pubis (Fig. 1.5). They extend laterally and attach to the arcus tendineus and levator ani muscle. Anteriorly they form the anterior pubourethral ligament which is an extension of the suspensory ligament of the clitoris and attaches near the external urethral meatus.[2,7] The pubourethral ligaments would seem to support the midurethral area. Their role in stress incontinence has been debated. Some authors have suggested that the posterior pubourethral ligaments are crucial for the support of the urethra and maintenance of continence during increases in abdominal pressure.[8] However, Delancey pointed out that the insertion of the pubourethral ligaments are actually below the bladder neck and distal to the region thought to be responsible for continence.[1] Weakness here would permit inferior and posterior movement of the midurethra, without displacement of the bladder neck.

As one extends proximally toward the bladder base, the anterior vaginal wall fascia is known as the pubocervical fascia (a condensation of perivesical and perivaginal fascia).[9] This fascia supports the bladder base to the lateral pelvic wall and arcus tendineus (Fig. 1.6). In bladder prolapse, or cystocele, this attachment may be weakened causing a laxity in the lateral support of the bladder to the pelvic side wall (lateral defect) or there may be a herniation of the bladder through a midline defect in the fascia itself (central defect).[10] Continuing proximally toward the cervix, the pubocervical fascia fuses with the paired car-

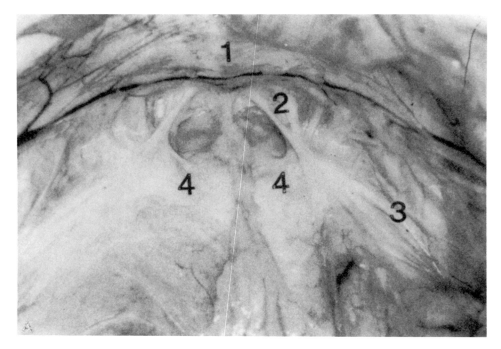

Fig. 1.5. Floor of the space of Retzius in an elderly female cadaver without pelvic prolapse. The entire space is covered with a continuous sheet of endopelvic fascia forming visible regional condensations. 1 = symphysis pubis; 2 = right posterior pubourethral complex; 3 = lateral condensation of endopelvic fascia forming right arcus tendinaeus fascia pelvis; 4 = condensation of the endopelvic fascia, which forms the whitish aponeurosis over the proximal urethra and internal vesical orifice. (From Mostwin, ref. 7, with permission.)

dinal ligaments. These ligaments extend from the lateral cervix to the arcus tendineus and with the uterosacral ligaments support the cervix and upper vagina over the levator plate. The cardinal ligaments also provide support to the base of the bladder as the fuse with the pubocervical fascia. In cases of uterine prolapse, the cardinal ligaments are lax displacing the pubocervical fascia laterally and predisposing to cystocele formation.[3]

Intrinsic and Extrinsic Urethral Sphincter in the Female

Equal in importance to the contribution of pelvic anatomy and support to urinary continence in the female are the intrinsic and external sphincteric mechanisms. Most of the intrinsic continence mechanism is in the midurethra.[11–13] The midurethra has been shown to be made up of five distinct layers[12,13] (Fig. 1.7). The innermost is the epithelial layer made up of transitional cells proximally and stratified squamous cells distally. The submucosa is next and has a significant contribution to the continence mechanism. It consists largely of a rich vascular sponge and is built out of loosely woven connective tissue infiltrated throughout by tiny smooth muscle bundles and an elaborate vascular plexus. The large and numerous veins are fed by many arterial-venous anastomoses and act to compress the mucosal folds and create a watertight closure.[13] Alteration of the arterial inflow to these venous channels has been shown to affect urethral pressure.[14,15] Beneath the sub-

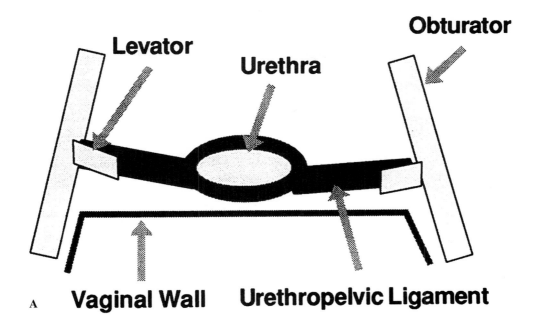

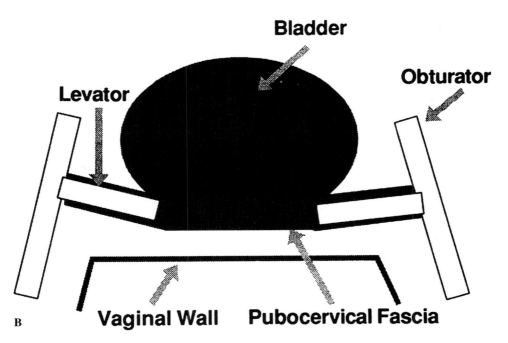

Fig. 1.6. Schematic cross-sectional view of **A:** the urethropelvic ligament and **B:** more proximally, the pubocervical fascia. From Nitti et al, ref. 3b, with permission.)

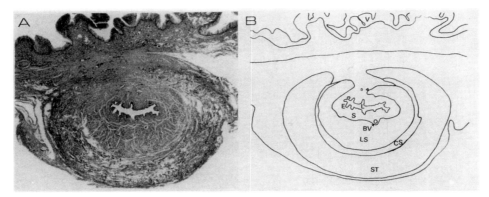

Fig. 1.7. A: Typical transverse section from midsection site of human female urethra. Reduced from ×8.2. **B:** Diagrammatic representation of section in part A to illustrate various tissue components seen. L = urethral lumen; E = urethral epithelium; S = submucosa; LS = longitudinal smooth muscle; CS = circular smooth muscle; BV = blood vessels; ST = striated muscle; V = vaginal epithelium. Gland tissue not shown. (From Carlile et al, ref. 12, with permission.)

mucosa are the muscle layers. All muscle layers are sparse toward the dorsal (vaginal) side of the urethra and thickest ventrally.[12,13] First are two layers of smooth muscle, the longitudinal inner and circular outer layer. Huisman considers these smooth muscle layers to be continuous with the musculature of the trigone and thus to be involved in micturition (but not continence) perhaps by maintaining the shape of the urethra.[13] However, the smooth muscle coat may help to maintain the "washer effect" of the submucosa by directing submucosal expansile pressures inward toward the mucosa, helping to maintain the mucosal seal.[9,16] The outer muscular layer is composed of striated muscle. Gosling and associates found a high concentration of slow-twitch fiber in this muscle layer and suggested a role in the maintenance of passive continence.[17]

Oelrich and Delancey further defined the anatomy of the extrinsic continence mechanism in the female.[1,2,11,18,19] By careful anatomic dissection, Oelrich identified three distinct muscles[18] (Fig. 1.8). The urethral sphincter is the striated muscle layer that surrounds the urethra for about 1.5 cm. As others have shown, in the adult this muscle is thick ventrally and thin or absent dorsally[12,13] (Fig. 1.7). Fibers are predominately oriented circularly and a few attach to the endopelvic fascia.[18] Distal to and continuous with the urethral sphincter is the compressor urethrae. It originates laterally and at the ischiopubic ramus. Near the urethra it is also continuous with the third muscle, the urethrovaginal sphincter. Fibers from the urethrovaginal sphincter originate in the vaginal wall. They encircle the urethra and vagina. The distal 20% of the urethra is devoid of muscle. The exact role of the striated urethral "sphincter" in the maintenance of urinary continence is debatable. Delancey has proposed that the three extrinsic muscles work together as a single unit to maintain constant urethral tone.[1] There may be a role for the compressor urethrae and urethrovaginal sphincter in elongation, compression, and retraction of the urethra.[18,19] Huisman, on the other hand, questioned the role of this striated muscle layer in continence.[13] McGuire has suggested that the external sphincter plays little role in the resistance of the urethra to changes in abdominal pressure, but rather is designed to resist changes in detrusor pressure (e.g., an unwanted detrusor contraction) through the spinal reflex.[20,21]

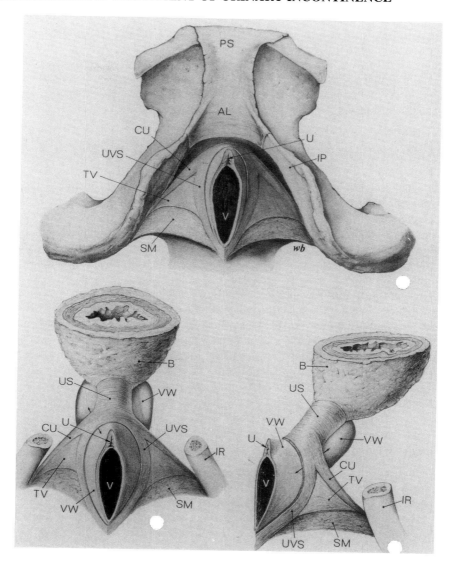

Fig. 1.8. Oblique view of the complete urogenital sphincter in the female. PS = pubic symphysis; AL = external anal; IP = ischiopubic ramus; B = bladder; US = urethral sphincter; VW = vaginal wall; CU = compressor urethrae muscle; TV = transverse vaginal muscle; UVS = urethrovaginal sphincter; SM = smooth muscle of urethrovaginal compartment; IR = ischial ramus. (From Oelrich, ref. 18, with permission.)

Summary

In summary, the function of the female bladder neck and urethra with respect to urinary continence is dependent on their anatomic position and support as well as intrinsic sphincter characteristics. Because these may change with childbirth and estrogen loss, incontinence is a common problem. Changes in the pelvic supporting structures result in downward displacement of the continence mechanism during increases in intra-abdominal pressure. More importantly, the increases in urethral resistance from the impact of the urethra on these supporting structures may also be lost, resulting in stress incontinence. In addition, the effective "mucosal seal" which is responsible for the intrinsic sphincteric nature of the urethra can also be affected by aging, estrogen loss, and pelvic surgery. Changes in any of the various layers of the urethral wall may result in decreased resistance and incontinence also.

ANATOMY OF MALE URINARY CONTINENCE

Unlike in the female, changes in the male bladder outlet with aging generally do not result in incontinence due to "outlet dysfunction". The most common sequela of aging affecting the male bladder outlet is obstruction from benign prostatic hyperplasia (BPH) or prostatic carcinoma. Although incontinence may ensue, it is usually due to bladder dysfunction which manifests as detrusor instability or to overflow. True sphincteric dysfunction usually only occurs as a result of trauma, prostatic surgery, or neurologic disease. The overwhelming majority of incontinence secondary to non-neurologic sphincter dysfunction in the male is postprostatectomy incontinence.

The male continence mechanism may be viewed as two functional urethral sphincters, the proximal and distal urethral sphincters. The proximal sphincteric mechanism is centered around the bladder neck but is functional from the bladder neck to the verumontanum.[22] It includes the "preprostatic sphincter," which consists of the extension of the circular bladder neck periurethral smooth muscle fibers into the prostatic urethra to the level of the verumontanum.[23,24] The distal urethral continence mechanism extends from the verumontanum, traverses the prostatic apex and ends at the perineal membrane. Each of these sphincters has its own unique function (Fig. 1.9).

Proximal Urethral Continence Mechanism

The bladder neck is made up of a complete circular collar of smooth muscle that surrounds the urethra proximal to the prostate. The exact origin of this muscle has been debated. Gosling, Dixon, and others feel that the bladder musculature has a separate origin, but merges with and is indistinguishable from the musculature of the prostatic capsule.[25–27] Others feel that the longitudinal muscle of the bladder base extends distally into the urethra.[28,29] Regardless of the exact origin of the smooth muscle of the proximal urethral sphincter (PUS), its sphincteric function is what is of most interest in the discussion of male continence. It has been suggested that this sphincteric function is provided by loops of smooth muscle acting in opposite directions: an outer horseshoe of smooth muscle with legs in a posterocephaled direction and an interdigitating inner semicircular horseshoe of trigonal muscle with legs in an anterocaudal direction. These loops may act in opposite directions to close the bladder neck during storage. The bladder neck opens when the two opposing loops relax as the detrusor muscle contracts.[30,31]

It is generally accepted that the PUS can maintain passive continence. It is normally competent when the detrusor is at rest but opens widely in association with a detrusor contraction.[22] Therefore, in a patient whose distal sphincter mechanism is nonfunctional, involuntary detrusor contractions will result in opening of the bladder neck and urinary incontinence.[32,33] In a stable bladder, an intact bladder neck alone can maintain urinary continence without a functional distal mechanism. While the PUS is certainly richly inner-

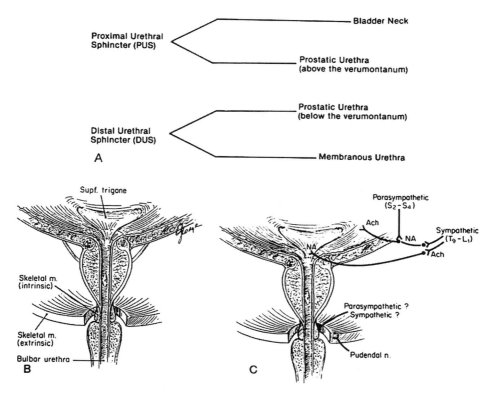

Fig. 1.9. A–C: Anatomy and innervation of the proximal and distal urethral sphincters. (From Hadley et al, ref. 27, with permission.)

vated by the sympathetic nervous system (see below), the mechanism of continence is not exclusively dependent on that innervation.[27,34,35] This is evidenced by studying patients who have had trauma which obliterates the sympathetic nervous system or operative sympathectomy.[34] These patients for the most part have a closed PUS and continence is probably due to spontaneous activity of smooth muscle and its arrangement around the bladder neck.[27]

Distal Urethral Continence Mechanism

The distal urethral sphincter (DUS) includes all of the anatomic structures of the urethra extending from the verumontanum, through the membranous urethra and ending at the perineal membrane. It consists of the following: (1) an inner layer of epithelial folds with an abundant vascular supply that contributes to urethral suppleness, allowing sufficient urethral coaptation from a minimal amount of pressure; (2) a middle layer composed of smooth muscle and elastic tissue; (3) an outer layer of intrinsic and extrinsic skeletal muscle.[27] Gosling has described the intrinsic skeletal muscle consisting of "slow-twitch" fibers which were felt to be innervated by the autonomic nervous system and are closely attached to the underlying urethra. These fibers maintain tonus for prolonged periods and are important in passive continence.[17,25] The outer or extrinsic layer of skeletal muscle, innervated by the pudendal nerve, consists of "fast-twitch" fibers and is similar to the sur-rounding pelvic floor muscles. It attaches to the urethra only on the posterior aspect and contributes minimally to passive continence, although voluntary contractions of this layer reinforce the DUS during straining and coughing and allow interruption of the urinary stream.[25] In contrast, Myers described the striated muscle of the DUS as a "horseshoe-shaped" muscle" that starts at the prostatic apex, remains mostly on the anterior and lateral surface of the membranous urethra and becomes thicker distally as the perineal membrane is approached.[36] At the level of the midmembranous urethra, the striated muscle can have more than three times the cross-sectional area of the urethra with its circumferential smooth muscle and scanty fibroelastic tissue.[36] A significant proportion of these striated muscle fibers are slow-twitch providing steady tonic compression of the urethra; the remainder are fast-twitch fibers.[17,37,38]

The levator ani musculature is the most distal portion of the pelvic diaphragm and is in close contact with the membranous and, in the male, prostatic urethra. The most distal portion of the levator ani is thought to provide lateral support to the membranous urethra, compression with contraction, and contributes to sudden cessation of voiding.[36] Most of the periurethral levator ani muscle has been shown to be slow-twitch fibers and may be related to their role in tonic support of the pelvic viscera. However, fast-twitch fibers are also present in the levator ani complex and are recruited to produce rapid, forceful occlusion of the urethra during sudden increases in intra-abdominal pressure.[17]

BLADDER MORPHOLOGY: RELATIONSHIP TO URINE STORAGE AND EMPTYING

The bladder may be divided into two parts, the body and the base.[39] The body consists of that portion above the ureteral orifices while the base encompasses the posterior trigone, deep detrusor, and anterior bladder wall.[39,40] A portion of the bladder base is continuous with the lower ureters. The superficial trigone is derived from the longitudinal muscle fibers of the intravesical ureter while fibers from Waldeyer's sheath form the deep trigone.[41] These fibers making up the trigone are superimposed on the detrusor as they make their way toward the bladder neck. This arrangement allows for the free efflux of urine from the ureters into the bladder and prevents reflux back into the ureter as the stretching of the trigone with progressive filling of the bladder increases resistance at the intravesical ureter. Similarly, during voiding with large increases in intravesical pressure, the contraction of the trigone completely closes the intravesical ureter.[41]

Once urine makes its way to the bladder it is important that it be stored at low pressures and effectively evacuated in a voluntary manner. On a structural level, the muscle cells of the bladder are arranged randomly in bundles lacking any architectural organization.[42] These muscle bundles have no discrete layers and continuously change planes freely inter-lacing with each other.[43] The spherical shape of the bladder as well as the viscoelastic properties of its components contribute to its excellent compliance allowing storage of pro-gressive volumes of urine at low pressure. The syncytial arrangement of muscle bundles, on the other hand, facilitates complete emptying of its contents.[40] Storage and evacuation of urine are further understood by considering the structure and interaction of the main components of the bladder: smooth muscle, interstitium, and intrinsic nerves. During stor-age, the intrinsic myogenic and elastic properties of the smooth muscle and interstitium (collagen and elastin) are responsible for compliance, while the interaction of smooth muscle and intrinsic nerves is responsible for bladder stability. To initiate emptying, intrinsic nerves initiate a contraction which is generated by smooth muscle cells and converted by the interstitium into a unitary contraction involving the entire detrusor.

In 1941 Bozler described two types of smooth muscle, multiunit and unitary.[44] Multiunit smooth muscle has a 1:1 ratio between nerve endings and muscle cells, whereas unitary smooth muscle has a much less extensive innervation and relies on gap junctions to propagate a contraction from one cell to another. The smooth muscle of the bladder seems to share characteristics of both types of smooth muscle. El Badawi and Schenk theorized a nearly 1:1 ratio whereas others argued for a considerably less than 1:1 ratio of nerve to muscle cells.[39,45] More recent ultrastructural studies by El Badawa showed that no portion of the bladder has exclusively a 1:1 ratio.[46] Wein and Barrett concluded that the bladder smooth muscle seems to possess both **multiunit** and unitary characteristics. However, there appears to be more properties of the **multiunit type,** "with some morphological substrates compatible with cell coupling and the capability of impulse propagation from cell to cell."[47] It is difficult to view bladder function strictly on a structural level. Further understanding of urine storage and evacuation requires knowledge of lower urinary tract neurophysiology.

NEUROPHYSIOLOGY OF URINE STORAGE AND MICTURITION

The autonomic and somatic nervous systems play a crucial role in lower urinary tract function. Normal voiding occurs when the bladder responds to threshold tension via its mechanoreceptors. In order that this does not occur randomly, central nervous system inhibitory and facilitatory pathways are involved in coordination of urine storage and micturition. In this section we will present a practical overview of this neurophysiology as it relates to the evaluation of voiding dysfunction and incontinence. The interested reader is referred to several recent reviews on the subject which present a more comprehensive discussion then can be included here.[40,48] Figure 10, adapted from deGroat, provides a working schematic to understand reflex pathways involved in micturition.[48a]

Central Innervation of the Lower Urinary Tract

The main function of the central nervous system is to facilitate and coordinate the various aspects of bladder filling, storage, and emptying. These functions are divided into spinal, pontine, and suprapontine centers.

The act of voiding is coordinated at the level of the brain stem specifically in the neurons of the pontine–mesencephalic gray matter or the pontine micturition center.[49–54] Micturition depends on a spinobulbospinal reflex relayed through this center, which receives input from the cerebral cortex, cerebellum, basal ganglia, thalamus, and hypothalamus. Much of the input from suprapontine centers appears to be inhibitory although there are some facilitory influences. The central facilitory areas are the anterior pons and the posterior hypothalamus, and the inhibitory areas include the cerebral cortex, basal ganglia, and cerebellum.[49–51,53,55–57] The cerebellum is also implicated in the maintenance of tone in the pelvic floor striated musculature and coordination between bladder contraction and periurethral striated muscle relaxation.[49–51] Since most of the suprapontine input to the pontine micturition center is inhibitory, interruption of this input (e.g. cerebrovascular accident, cerebral atrophy, Parkinson's disease, brain tumor or trauma) often results in uncontrolled detrusor activity, or hyperreflexia. These uninhibited detrusor contractions result in urinary frequency, urgency, and urge incontinence.

Spinal Cord

Afferents

The two areas of the spinal cord responsible for transmitting afferent input from the lower urinary tract are the lateral spinothalamic tracts and the posterior columns. The lateral spinothalamic tracts contain ascending routes responsible for transmitting bladder sensation and triggering voiding. Sectioning of these tracts results in loss of bladder sensation and voiding. Ascending sensory stimuli include exteroceptive sensory impulses such as pain, temperature, and touch and are generated in the urothelium.[50,51,58] Proprioceptive sensory impulses generated in bladder muscle and periurethral striated muscle travel in the posterior columns.[50,51,58]

Efferents

The pontine micturition center controls efferent input to the bladder and external sphincter via two separate regions. The medial region is responsible for motor input to the detrusor muscle via the reticulospinal tracts to the sacral intermediolateral cell groups, which contain preganglionic parasympathetic neurons that form the motor supply of the detrusor.[30,40] Electrical stimulation of this region results in a prompt decrease in pelvic floor EMG and urethral pressure followed by an increase in detrusor pressure. The lateral region has specific projections via the corticospinal tracts to the nucleus of Onuf in the sacral cord which contains motor neurons innervating the pelvic floor including the urethral and anal sphincters.[30,40] Electrical stimulation of this region results in a rapid increase in urethral pressure and pelvic floor EMG but little increase in intravesical pressure.

Peripheral Innervation

Coordinated voiding depends on integrated autonomic (sympathetic and parasympathetic) and somatic innervation to the lower urinary tract. Parasympathetic efferent input to the bladder arises from the intermediolateral cell column of S2–4 and travels as preganglionic fibers via the *pelvic nerve* to the pelvic plexus located on both sides of the rectum from which postganglionic fibers innervate the bladder.[40,46,48,50,59–61] Efferent sympathetic nerves to the bladder and urethra arise from the intermediolateral cell column of T10–L2 as preganglionic fibers that travel to ganglia located in the superior hypogastric plexus, from which arises the *hypogastric nerve* which contains the postganglionic sympathetic efferents to the bladder and urethra.[40,48,46,62]

Both the pelvic and hypogastric nerves as well as the pudendal nerve also convey afferent fibers from the bladder and urethra to the dorsal columns of the lumbosacral spinal cord.[46,48–50,59–61] Afferent terminals are located in the submucosa and muscularis and travel in the pelvic, pudendal, and hypogastric nerves. Most afferent axons terminate as free nerve endings without specialized receptors except for sparse pacinian corpuscles.[60] There is some specialization of afferent sensations, however. Different sensations are detected by specialized receptors and travel along different nerves: afferent fibers detecting the sensation of bladder distension travel in the pelvic nerves; afferents from mechanoreceptors travel along the hypogastric nerve; nociceptor afferents travel along both pelvic and hypogastric nerves. Afferents from the striated sphincter and urethra transmit sensation of urethral wall distension, urine passage, temperature, and pain and travel along the pudendal nerve.[63,64] According to cat studies, afferents detecting the sensation of distension are more prominent in muscle than in the submucosa; afferents traveling in the hypogastric nerve detecting sensations of pain, conscious touch, and distension are most prominent in the trigone and anterior bladder neck region.[60]

The innervation of the striated muscle of the external urethral sphincter is controversial. It is most probably primarily somatic by the pudendal nerve, which contains motor axons from Onuf's nucleus located in the second to fourth segments of the sacral spinal cord.[40,46,61,65–70] Some authors feel that both the intrinsic and extrinsic components are innervated by somatic fibers.[68] Others think that the intrinsic component is innervated by both somatic and autonomic fibers.[46,62,71,72] Neuroinnervation of the lower urinary tract is summarized in Fig. 1.10.

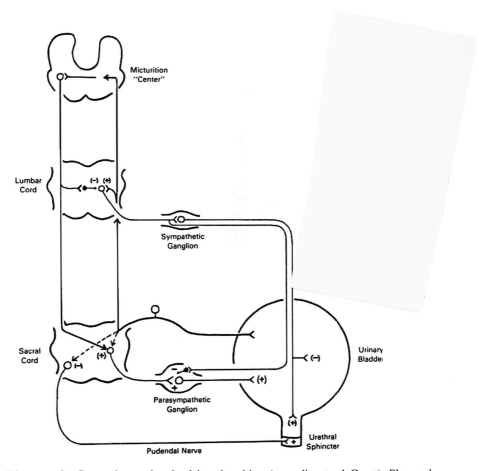

Fig. 1.10. Diagram of reflex pathways involved in micturition (according to deGroat). Plus and minus signs indicate, respectively, exicitatory and inhibitory synaptic actions. The connection of the pontine micturition center to the cerebral cortex and other suprapontine areas is not pictured. (From deGroat and Booth, ref. 48a, with permission.)

Neuroreceptors

Classically, peripheral innervation of the bladder is thought to be parasympathetic via the pelvic nerve and innervation to the bladder neck and proximal sphincter is felt to be predominately sympathetic via the hypogastric nerve. Numerous authors have described an abundant cholinergic innervation of the bladder and less dense cholinergic innervation of the bladder neck and proximal urethra in both sexes.[69,73] On the other hand, adrenergic innervation of the human bladder is sparse but there is an increase as the area of the trigone is approached.[31,63,67,73–75] The male bladder neck and preprostatic urethra have been shown to possess a rich adrenergic innervation, while the human female bladder neck and proximal urethra contain relatively few adrenergic nerves.[48,63,69] The prostatic urethra in the human male contains a high concentration of α_1-adrenergic receptors, which have been shown to mediate contraction of prostatic smooth muscle and have a significant role in the pathophysiology and management of benign prostatic hyperplasia.[76–81] The prostate contains fewer cholinergic receptors, which do not appear to be involved in prostatic muscle contraction.[77]

In addition to adrenergic and cholinergic receptors, a variety of nonadrenergic, noncholinergic receptors have been implicated in lower urinary tract function. Neuropeptides such as neuropeptide Y, substance P, vasoactive intestinal peptide (VIP), enkephalin, cholecystokinin and somatostatin have been found to have various inhibitory and facilitory effects on cholinergic transmission at the level of the pelvic ganglia and plexus and bladder.[40,82–86] γ-Aminobutyric acid (GABA) may have central as well as peripheral influence. It has been shown to inhibit excitatory efferent transmission in the pelvic ganglia.[40,87] Serotonin (5-HT) is also involved in peripheral control of the lower urinary tract and although it has been shown to be both excitatory and inhibitory, its predominant effect seems to be to inhibit cholinergic transmission in the pelvic ganglia.[40,88]

Voiding Dysfunction and Neurologic Disease

Storage and evacuation of urine depends on neural integration at the peripheral, spinal cord, and central levels. Normally, bladder distension will cause low level firing of afferent nerves. This will cause reflex inhibitory response to the bladder via the hypogastric nerve and stimulatory response to the external sphincter from the pudendal nerve. With further distension myelinated A-delta fiber afferents are activated. Afferents travel up the spinal cord to the pontine micturition center. Here central input, mostly inhibitory, is received from suprapontine centers. If voiding is not desired, the voiding reflex can be interrupted. If voiding is desired, efferent output to the pelvic plexus at S2–4 via the spinal cord is initiated. Ultimately the stimulatory message is sent to the bladder via the pelvic nerve. At the same time inhibitory messages are sent to the hypogastric and pudendal pathways to allow for relaxation of the sphincter mechanisms and coordinated voiding (Fig. 1.10).

Pathologic processes at each level of innervation must be considered when evaluating neurogenic voiding dysfunction. For example, suprapontine lesions (e.g., cerebral atrophy, cerebrovascular accident, brain tumor) will cause a loss of inhibitory input to the pontine micturition center and subsequent uninhibited bladder contractions. Sphincter reflexes are not affected and coordinated uninhibited voiding can result.[89,90] Suprasacral spinal cord lesions will also result in loss of supraspinal input, however the complexity of the resulting voiding dysfunction will depend on the level and completeness of the lesion. Also input to the sphincters may be disrupted resulting in detrusor–sphincter dyssynergia (DSD). A complete spinal cord lesion will result in the development of a spinal micturition reflex. Unmylenated C-fiber afferents excite sacral neurons and trigger a bladder contraction.[91] In addition there is incomplete relaxation of the external sphincter (DSD), resulting in a contraction against a closed outlet with subsequent incontinence, retention, and eventual loss of bladder compliance. If the lesion is above the level of the sympathetic ganglia (T10–L1) detrusor–internal sphincter dyssynergia may also occur. Lesions of the sacral cord may present with various degrees of upper or lower motor neuron type bladders, ranging from the hyperreflexic suprasacral type, to the areflexic infrasacral type. The external sphincter is similarly and variably affected ranging from nonfunctional to DSD. Infrasacral cord and peripheral nerve lesions generally result in loss of sensation and contractility, leading to a large, supercompliant, areflexic bladder. The external sphincter may also be deficient of contractility and tone.

REFERENCES

1. Delancey JO: Structure and function of the continence mechanism relative to stress incontinence. *Problems in Urology* 5(1):1–10, 1991.

2. Delancey JO: Pubovesical ligament: a separate structure from the urethral supports ("pubo-urethral ligaments"). *Neurourol Urodyn* 8:53–61, 1989.

3. Raz S, Little NA, Juma S: Female urology. In Walsh PC, Retik AB, Stamey TA, et al (eds): *Campbell's Urology*, ed 6. Philadelphia, WB Saunders, 1992, pp 2782–2828.

3a. Klutke C, Golomb J, Barbaric Z, et al: The anatomy of stress incontinence: magnetic resonance imaging of the female bladder neck and urethra. *J Urol* 143:563–566, 1990.

3b. Nitti VW, Bregg KG, Raz S: Surgical management of incontinence in elderly women. In O'Donnell PA: *Geriatric Urology*. Boston, Little Brown, 1994, pp 239–263.

4. Raz S, Sussman EM, Erikson DE, et al: The Raz bladder neck suspension: results in 206 patients. *J Urol* 148:845–850, 1992.

5. Raz S, Klutke CG, Golub J: Four-corner bladder and urethral suspension for moderate cystocele. *J Urol* 142:712–715, 1989.

6. Raz S, Little NA, Juma S, et al: Repair of severe anterior vaginal wall prolapse (Grade IV Cystourethrocele). *J Urol* 146:988–992, 1991.

7. Mostwin JL: Current concepts of female pelvic anatomy and physiology. *Urol Clin North Am* 18:175–195, 1991.

8. Zacharin RF: The anatomic supports of the female urethra. *Obstet Gynecol* 32:754–759, 1968.

9. Staskin DR, Zimmern PE, Hadley HR, et al: The pathophysiology of stress incontinence. *Urol Clin North Am* 12:271–278, 1985.

10. Raz S, Sussman EM, Erikson DE: Vaginal repair of high grade cystocele. *Contemp Urol* 3(5):80–94, 1991.

11. Delancey JO: Correlative study of paraurethral anatomy. *Obstet Gynecol* 68:91–97, 1986.

12. Carlile A, Davies I, Rigby A, et al: Age changes in the human female urethra: a morphometric study. *J Urol* 139:532–535, 1988.

13. Huisman AB: Aspects on the anatomy of the female urethra with special relation to urinary continence. *Contrib Gynec Obstet* 10:1–31, 1983.

14. Raz S, Caine M, Zeigler M: The vascular component in the production of intraurethral pressure. *J Urol* 108:93–96, 1972.

15. Rud T, Anderson KE, Asmussen M, et al: Factors maintaining the intraurethral pressure in women. *Invest Urol* 17:343–347, 1980.

16. Raz S: Vaginal approach to urinary incontinence. In Glenn JF: *Urologic Surgery,* ed 4. Philadelphia, Lippincott, 1991, pp 790–804.

17. Gosling JA, Dixon JS, Critchley OD, et al: A comparative study of the human external sphincter and periurethral levator ani muscles. *Br J Urol* 53:35–41, 1981.

18. Oelrich TM: The striated urogenital sphincter muscle in the female. *Anat Rec* 205:223–232, 1983.

19. Delancey JO: Structural aspects of the extrinsic continence mechanism. *Obstet Gynecol* 72:296–301, 1988.

20. McGuire EJ, Appell RA: Collagen injection for the dysfunctional urethra. *Comtemp Urol* 3(Sept.):11–19, 1991.

21. McGuire EJ: Collagen injection treatment of incontinence. American Urological Association—Pelvic Reconstruction and Voiding Dysfunction, March 4–6, 1994, pp 141–148.

22. Turner Warwick R: The sphincter mechanisms: their relation to prostatic enlargement and its treatment. In Hinman F Jr: *Benign Prostatic Hypertrophy.* New York, Springer-Verlag, 1983, pp 809–828.

23. McNeal JE: The prostate and prostatic urethra: a morphologic synthesis. *J Urol* 107:1008, 1972.

24. Blacklock NJ: Surgical anatomy of the prostate. In Williams DI, Chisholm GD: *Scientific Foundations of Urology.* London, William Heinemann, 1976, pp 113–125.

25. Gosling J: Symposium on clinical urodynamics. *Urol Clin North Am* 6:31–38, 1979.

26. Dixon J, Gosling J: Structure and innervation of human bladder. In Torrens M, Morrison JFB: *The Physiology of the Lower Urinary Tract.* Berlin, Springer–Verlag, 1987, pp 3–20.

27. Hadley HR, Zimmern P, Raz S: The treatment of male urinary incontinence. In Walsh PC, Retik AB, Stamey TA, et al (eds): *Campbell's Urology,* ed 5. Philadelphia, WB Saunders, 1986, pp 2658–2679.

28. Hutch JA, Rambo OA: A new theory of the anatomy of the internal urinary sphincter and the physiology of micturition III. Anatomy of the urethra. *J Urol* 97:696, 1967.

29. Tanagho EA: The ureterovesical junction: anatomy and physiology. In Chrisholm GD, Williams DI: *Scientific Foundations of Urology.* Chicago, Year Book Medical Publishers, 1982, pp 295–405.

30. Bradley WE: Innervation of the male urinary bladder. *Urol Clin North Am* 5:279–293, 1978.

31. Bradley WE: Physiology of the urinary bladder. In Walsh PC, Retik AB, Stamey TA, et al (eds): *Campbell's Urology,* ed 5. Philadelphia, WB Saunders, 1986, pp 129–185.

32. Turner Warwick R: Clinical problems associated with urodynamic abnormalities. In Lutzeyer W, Melchior H: *Urodynamics.* Berlin, Springer-Verlag, 1972, pp 237–263.

33. Turner Warwick R: Clinical urodynamics. *Urol Clin North Am* 6:13–30, 51–54, 63–70, 171–198, 1975.

34. Nordling J: Influence of the sympathetic nervous system on the lower urinary tract in man. *Neurourol Urodyn* 2:3, 1982.

35. Crowley JA, Dixon JS, London RG: The anatomic innervation of the human male and female bladder neck and proximal urethra. *J Urol* 118:302–305, 1977.

36. Myers RP: Male urethral sphincter anatomy and radical prostatectomy. *Urol Clin North Am* 18:211–227, 1991.

37. Schroeder HD, Reske-Nielsen E: Fiber types in the striated and anal sphincter. *Acta Neuropath* 60:278–282, 1983.

38. Yalla SO, Dibenedetto M, Fam BA, et al: Striated sphincter participation in distal passive urinary continence mechanisms: studies in male subjects deprived of primary sphincter mechanism. *J Urol* 122:655–660, 1979.

39. El Badawi A, Schenk EA: Dual innervation of the mammalian urinary bladder: a histochemical study of the distributions of cholinergic and adrenergic nerves. *Am J Anat* 119:405–427, 1966.

40. Steers WD: Physiology of the urinary bladder. In Walsh PC, Retik AB, Stamey TA, et al (eds): *Campbell's Urology,* ed 6. Philadelphia, WB Saunders, 1992, pp 142–176.

41. Tanagho EA: Anatomy of the lower urinary tract. In Walsh PC, Retik AB, Stamey TA, et al (eds): *Campbell's Urology,* ed 6. Philadelphia, WB Saunders, 1992, pp 40–69.

42. Donker PJ, Droes JP, and Van Adler BM: Anatomy of the musculature and innervation of the bladder and urethra. In Chrisholm GD, Williams DI. *Scientific Foundations of Urology.* Chicago, Year Book Medical Publishers, 1982, pp 404–441.

43. Hunter deW T Jr: A new concept of the urinary bladder musculature. *J Urol* 71:695–704, 1954.

44. Bozler E: Action potentials and conduction of excitation in smooth muscle. *Biol Symp* 3:95, 1941.

45. Raezer DM, Wein AJ, Jacobowitz D, et al: Autonomic innervation of canine urinary bladder; cholinergic and adrenergic contributions and interaction of sympathetic and parasympathetic systems in bladder function. *Urology* 2:211–221, 1973.

46. El Badawi A: Neuromorphologic basis of vesicourethral function. I. Histochemistry, ultrastructure and function of intrinsic nerves of the bladder and urethra. *Neurourol Urodyn* 1:3, 1982.

47. Wein AJ, Barrett DM: *Voiding Function and Dysfunction.* Chicago, Yearbook Medical Publishers, 1988, pp 22–31.

48. Wein AJ, Levin RM, Barnett DM: Voiding function and dysfunction. In Gillenwater JY, Grayhack JT, Howards SS, et al (eds): *Adult and Pediatric Urology,* ed 5. Chicago, Yearbook Medical Publishers, 1991, pp 933–1100.

48a. deGroat WC, Booth AM: Physiology of the urinary bladder and urethra. *Ann Intern Med,* 92 (part 2):312–315, 1980.

49. Bradley WE, Timm GW, Scott FB: Innervation of the detrusor muscle and urethra. *Urol Clin North Am* 1:3–27, 1974.

50. Bradley WE, Sundin T: The physiology and pharmacology of urinary tract dysfunction. *Clin Neuropharmacol* 5:131–158, 1982.

51. Bhatia NN, Bradley WE: Neuroanatomy and physiology: innervation of the urinary tract. In Raz S: *Female Urology.* Philadelphia, WB Saunders, 1983, pp 12–32.

52. deGroat WC, Ryall RW: Reflexes to sacral parasympathetic neurons concerned with micturition in the cat. *J Physiol* 200:87–108, 1969.

53. Carlsson CA: The supraspinal control of the urinary bladder. *Acta Pharmacol Toxicol* 43(suppl 2):8–12, 1978.

54. de Groat WC, Steers WD: Autonomic regulation of the urinary bladder and sexual organs. In Loewy AD, Spyer KM: *Central Regulation of the Autonomic Functions.* Oxford, Oxford University Press, 1990, pp 313–333.

55. Tang PC: Levels of the brainstem and diencephalon controlling micturition reflex. *J Neurophysiol* 18:583–595, 1955.

56. Tang PC, Ruth TC: Localization of brainstem and diencephalic areas controlling the micturition reflex. *J Comp Neurol* 106:213–231, 1956.

57. Nathan PW: The central nervous connections of the bladder. In Williams DI, Chisholm GD: *Scientific Foundations of Urology.* Chicago, Yearbook Medical Publishers, 1976, vol 2, pp 51–58.

58. Bradley WE, Scott FB: Physiology of the urinary bladder. In Walsh PC, Retik AB, Stamey TA, et al (eds): *Campbell's Urology,* ed 5. Philadelphia, WB Saunders, 1986, pp 87–124.

59. Bors E, Comarr AE: *Neurological Urology.* Baltimore, University Park Press, 1971.

60. Fletcher TF, Bradley WE: Neuroanatomy of the bladder-urethra. *J Urol* 119:153–160, 1978.

61. El Badawi A: Autonomic muscular innervation of the vesical outlet and its role in micturition. In Hinman F Jr: *Benign Prostatic Hypertrophy.* Berlin, Springer-Verlag, 1983, pp 330–348.

62. Norlen L: Influence of the sympathetic nervous system on the lower urinary tract and its clinical implications. *Neurourol Urodyn* 1:129, 1982.

63. Kaneko S, Minami K, Yachiku S, et al: Bladder neck dysfunction: the effect of the adrenergic agent phentolamine on bladder neck dysfunction and a fluorescent histochemical study of bladder neck smooth muscle. *Invest Urol* 18:212–218, 1980.

64. de Groat WC, Kawatani M: Neural control of the urinary bladder: possible relationship between peptidergic inhibitory mechanisms and detrusor instability. *Neurourol Urodyn* 4:285–300, 1985.

65. McKenna K, Nadelhaft I: The organization of the pudendal nerve in the male and female cat. *J Comp Neurol* 248:532–549, 1985.

66. Tanagho EA, Schmidt RA, Gomes de Aranjo C: Urinary striated sphincter: what is its nerve supply? *Urology* 20:415–417, 1982.

67. Morita T, Nishizawa O, Noto H, et al: Pelvic nerve innervation of the external sphincter of urethra as suggested by urodynamic and horseradish studies. *J Urol* 131:591–595, 1984.

68. Gosling JA, Chilton CP: The structure of the bladder and urethra in relation to function. *Urol Clin North Am* 6:31–38, 1979.

69. Gosling JA, Chilton CP: The anatomy of the bladder, urethra and pelvic floor. In Mundy AR, Stephenson TP, Wein AJ. *Urodynamics, Principles, Practice and Applications.* London, Churchill Livingston, 1984, pp 3–13.

70. Sakuta M, Nakanishi T, Toyokura Y: Anal muscle electromyography difference in amyotrophic lateral sclerosis and Shy-Drager syndrome. *Neurology,* 28:1289–1292, 1978.

71. El Badawi A, Schenk SA: A new theory of the innervation of bladder musculature. III. Innervation of the vesicourethral junction and external urethral sphincter. *J Urol* 111:613–615, 1974.

72. El Badawi A, Atta MA: Ultrastructure of vesicourethral innervation: IV Evidence for somatomotor plus autonomic innervation of the pelvic rhabdosphincter. *Neurourol Urodyn* 4:23–36, 1985.

73. Kluck P: The autonomic innervation of the human urinary bladder, bladder neck, urethra: a histochemical study. *Anat Rec* 198:439–443, 1980.

74. Sundin T, Dahlstrom A, Norlen L, et al: The sympathetic innervation and adrenoreceptor function of the human lower urinary tract in the normal state and after parasympathetic denervation. *Invest Urol* 14:322–328, 1977.

75. Benson GS, McConnell JA, Wood JG: Adrenergic innervation of the human bladder body. *J Urol* 122:189–191, 1979.

76. Lepor H, Shapiro E: Characterization of alpha1 adrenergic receptors in human benign prostatic hyperplasia. *J Urol* 132:1226–1229, 1984.

77. Hedlund H, Andersson KE, Larsson B: Alpha-adrenoceptors and muscarinic receptors in the isolated human prostate. *J Urol* 134:1291–1298, 1985.

78. Shapiro E, Lepor H: Alpha1 adrenergic receptors in canine lower genitourinary tissues: inshight into development and function. *J Urol* 138:979–983, 1987.

79. Gup DI, Shapiro E, Baumann M, et al: Autonomic receptors in human prostate adenomas. *J Urol* 143:179–185, 1990.

80. Chapple CR, Aubry ML, James S, et al: Characterization of human prostatic adrenoceptors using pharmacology receptor binding and localisation. *Br J Urol* 63:487–496, 1989.

81. Lepor H, Gup DI, Baumann M, et al: Comparison of alpha1 adrenoceptors in the prostate capsule of men with symptomatic and asymptomatic benign prostatic hyperplasia. *Br J Urol* 67:493–498, 1991.

82. deGroat WC, Kawatani M, Booth AC: Enkephalinergic modulation of cholinergic transmission in the parasympathetic ganglia of the cat urinary bladder. In Hanin I: *Dynamics of Cholinergic* Function. New York, Plenum, 1986, pp 1007–1017.

83. deGroat WC, Kawatani M, Hisamitsu T, et al: Neural control of micturition: the role of neuropeptides. *J Auton Nerv Syst* (suppl): 369, 1986.

84. Gu J, Blank MA, Huang WM, et al: Neuropeptide containing nerves in human urinary bladder. *Urology* 24:353–357, 1984.

85. Kawatani M, Ratigliano M, deGroat WM: Selective facilitatory effects of vasoactive intestinal polypeptide on muscarinic mechanisms in sympathetic and parasympathetic ganglia of the cat. In Hanin I: *Dynamics of Cholinergic Function.* New York, Plenum, 1986, pp 1057–1065.

86. Kawatani M, Shioda A, Nakai Y, et al: Ultrastructural analysis of enkephalinergic terminal in the parasympathetic ganglia innervating the urinary bladder of the cat. *J Comp Neurol* 188:181–191, 1989.

87. deGroat WC, Booth AC: The effects of glycine, GABA, and strychnine on sacral parasympathetic preganglionic neurons. *Brain Res* 18:542, 1970.

88. Akasu T, Hasuo H, Tokimasa T: Activation of 5-HT$_3$ receptor subtypes causes rapid excitation of rabbit parasympathetic neurons. *Br J Pharmacol* 91:453–455, 1987.

89. Blaivas JG, Singa HP, Zayed AAH, et al: Detrusor-external sphincter-dyssynergia. *J Urol* 125:542–544, 1981.

90. Blaivas JG: The neurophysiology of normal micturition: a clinical study of 550 patients. *J Urol* 127:958–963, 1982.

91. deGroat WC, Nadelhaft I, Milne RJ, et al: Organization of the sacral parasympathetic reflex pathways to the urinary bladder and large intestine. *J Auton Nerv Syst* 3:135, 1981.

2

Classification, Diagnostic Evaluation, and Treatment Overview

Jerry G. Blaivas
Dianne M. Heritz

INTRODUCTION AND TERMINOLOGY

Urinary incontinence is the involuntary loss of urine. The term denotes a symptom, a sign, and a condition. The symptom is the complaint of involuntary urine loss. The sign is the objective demonstration of urine loss and the condition is the underlying pathophysiology.[1]

Incontinence may be urethral or extraurethral. Extraurethral incontinence is caused by urinary fistula or ectopic ureter. Urethral incontinence is due to either bladder abnormalities or sphincter abnormalities (Table 2.1). Cognitive abnormalities and physical immobility do not directly cause urinary incontinence but may be considered important cofactors in the genesis of symptoms.

Bladder abnormalities causing urinary incontinence are (1) detrusor overactivity and (2) low bladder compliance. *Detrusor overactivity* is a generic term for involuntary detrusor contractions. *Detrusor hyperreflexia* denotes involuntary detrusor contractions which are due to neurologic conditions. *Detrusor instability* denotes involuntary detrusor contractions that are not due to neurologic disorders.

Low bladder compliance describes an abnormal pressure/volume relationship wherein there is a high incremental rise in detrusor pressure during bladder filling.

Sphincter abnormalities are different in men and women. In men, sphincteric incontinence is due to either neurologic impairment or anatomic disruption after prostatic surgery or urethral trauma. In women there are two generic types of sphincteric incontinence—

TABLE 2.1. Conditions Causing Urinary Incontinence

Bladder Abnormalities	*Sphincter Abnormalities*
Detrusor overactivity	Urethral hypermobility
Detrusor instability	Intrinsic sphincter deficiency
Detrusor hyperreflexia	
Low bladder compliance	
Urinary fistula	

urethral hypermobility and intrinsic sphincter deficiency. In urethral hypermobility, the basic abnormality is a weakness of the pelvic floor. During increases in abdominal pressure there is rotational descent of the vesical neck and proximal urethra. If the urethra opens concomitantly, stress urinary incontinence ensues. Urethral hypermobility is often present in women who are not incontinent. Thus, the mere presence of urethral hypermobility is not sufficient to make a diagnosis of a sphincter abnormality unless incontinence is also demonstrated.

Intrinsic sphincteric deficiency denotes an intrinsic malfunction of the urethral sphincter itself. It is characterized by an open vesical neck at rest, a low leak point pressure and is usually the result of previous incontinence surgery or a neurologic lesion involving the thoracolumbar outflow.

Urethral hypermobility and intrinsic sphincter deficiency may coexist in the same patient. At the present time there are no well-defined objective methods to distinguish the two, but the abdominal leak point pressure, as discussed below, offers great promise.

Overflow incontinence is a descriptive term which denotes leakage of urine associated with urinary retention. The actual urine loss is caused by either sphincteric abnormalities or detrusor overactivity.

Another classification of stress incontinence in women, complementary to the one cited above, is based on anatomic and radiographic appearances.[2]

Type O SUI—The patient complains of a typical history of stress incontinence, but no urinary leakage is demonstrated during the clinical and urodynamic investigation. At videourodynamic study, the vesical neck and proximal urethra are closed at rest and situated at or above the inferior margin of the symphysis pubis. During stress the vesical neck and proximal urethra descend and open, assuming an anatomic configuration identical to that seen in Type I and II SUI. Failure to demonstrate incontinence is probably due to momentary voluntary contraction of the external urethral sphincter during the examination.

Type I SUI—The vesical neck is closed at rest and situated above the inferior margin of the symphysis. During stress the vesical neck and proximal urethra open, but there is minimal descent (less than 2 cm). Urinary incontinence is apparent during periods of increased abdominal pressure. There is little or no cystocele.

Type IIA—The vesical neck is closed at rest and situated above the inferior margin of the symphysis pubis. During stress the vesical neck and proximal urethra open and there is rotational descent characteristic of a cystourethrocele. Urinary incontinence is apparent during periods of increased intra-abdominal pressure.

Type IIB—The vesical neck is closed at rest and situated at or below the inferior margin of the symphysis pubis. During stress there may or may not be further descent, but the urethra opens and incontinence ensues.

Type III—The vesical neck and proximal urethra are open at rest in the absence of a detrusor contraction. The proximal urethra no longer functions as a sphincter. There is obvious urinary leakage which may be gravitational in nature or associated with minimal increases in intravesical pressure.

Type III SUI is the classic picture of intrinsic sphincter deficiency. We believe that Type I SUI is the earliest manifestation of intrinsic sphincter deficiency.

SYMPTOMS, SIGNS, AND CONDITIONS CAUSING INCONTINENCE (Table 2.2)

Urge incontinence—The symptom is incontinence associated with a sudden uncontrollable desire to void (urgency). The sign is the observation of involuntary urinary loss from the urethra synchronous with an uncontrollable urge to void. The condition is due to involuntary detrusor contraction. However, involuntary detrusor contractions are demonstrable at cystometry in only about 50–60% of patients who complain of urge incontinence. We believe that this is because the cystometrogram (CMG) is not sensitive enough.

Stress incontinence—The symptom is incontinence which occurs during coughing, sneezing, or physical exertion such as sport activities, sudden changes of position, etc. The sign is the observation of loss of urine from the urethra synchronous with straining, coughing, sneezing, or physical exertion. The condition is due to sphincter abnormalities or detrusor overactivity provoked by such physical activity. The latter condition is called *stress hyperreflexia.*

Unconscious incontinence—The symptom unconscious incontinence is incontinence which is unaccompanied by either urge or stress. The sign is the observation of loss of urine without patient awareness of urge or stress. The condition may be caused by detrusor overactivity, sphincter abnormalities, overflow, or extraurethral incontinence.

Continuous leakage—The symptom is the complaint of a continuous loss of urine. The sign is the observation of continuous urinary loss. The condition may be caused by sphincter abnormalities or extraurethral incontinence.

Nocturnal enuresis—The symptom is incontinence which occurs during sleep. The condition may be caused by a sphincter abnormality, detrusor overactivity, or extraurethral incontinence.

Postvoid dribble—The symptom is a dribbling incontinence which occurs immediately after voiding. The sign is the observation of such dribbling, but the condition underlying postvoid dribble has not been adequately defined. It is thought to be due to retained urine in the urethra distal to the sphincter in men. In women it may be caused by retained urine in the vagina or in a urethral diverticula.

DIAGNOSTIC EVALUATION

Diagnostic evaluation of urinary incontinence begins with a history, physical examination, and urinalysis and culture. Positive urine cultures should be treated with culture-specific antibiotics, but patients with persistent bacteriuria or recurrent infections may require invasive testing while on antibiotics. Hematuria should be fully evaluated. The history may be supplemented by a questionnaire. Micturition diaries and pad tests are important adjuncts which should be part of the routine evaluation.

TABLE 2.2. Symptoms, Signs, and Conditions Causing Urinary Incontinence

Symptom	Condition	Medical/Surgical Causes
Urge incontinence	Detrusor overactivity	1) Idiopathic 2) Neurogenic 3) Urinary tract infection 4) Bladder cancer 5) Outlet obstruction
Stress incontinence	1) Sphincter hypermobility 2) Intrinsic sphincter deficiency	1) Pelvic floor relaxation 2) Prior urethral, bladder, or pelvic surgery 3) Neurogenic
Unaware incontinence	1) Detrusor overactivity 2) Sphincter abnormality 3) Extraurethral incontinence	1) Idiopathic 2) Neurogenic 3) Prior urethral, bladder, or pelvic surgery 4) Vesico-, uretero-, or urethrovaginal fistula 5) Ectopic ureter
Continuous leakage	1) Sphincter abnormality 2) Impaired detrusor contractility 3) Extraurethral incontinence	1) Neurogenic 2) Prior urethral, bladder, or pelvic surgery 3) Ectopic ureter 4) Urinary/vaginal fistula
Nocturnal enuresis	1) Sphincter abnormality 2) Detrusor overactivity	1) Idiopathic 2) Neurogenic 3) Outlet obstruction
Postvoid dribble	Postsphincteric collection of urine	1) Idiopathic 2) Urethral diverticulum
Extraurethral incontinence	1) Vesico-, uretero-, or urethrovaginal fistula 2) Ectopic ureter	1) Trauma; surgical, obstetrical 2) Congenital

The sine qua non for a precise diagnosis is that the urinary incontinence is actually witnessed by the examiner. It makes little difference whether the urinary loss is demonstrated during physical examination, at cystoscopy, cystometry or by x-ray; the observations and measurements of an astute clinician are sufficient to arrive at the correct diagnosis in the majority of patients. In doubtful cases, videourodynamics is usually definitive.

UROLOGIC HISTORY

The history begins with a detailed account of the precise nature of the patient's symptoms. When more than one symptom is present, the patient's assessment of the relative severity of each should be noted. The patient should be asked how often he or she urinates during the day and what is the longest he or she can comfortably go between urinations. Does the patient void because of a severe urge or is it merely out of convenience or an attempt to prevent incontinence? The severity of incontinence should be graded. Is it just a few drops or does it saturate the outer clothing? Are protective pads worn? Do they become saturated? How often are they changed? Is the patient aware of the act of incontinence or does he/she just find himself/herself wet? Is there a sense of urgency first? If so, how long can micturition be postponed? Does urge incontinence occur? Does stress incontinence occur during coughing, sneezing, rising from a sitting to standing position or only during heavy physical exercise? If the incontinence is associated with stress, is urine lost only for an instant during the stress or is there uncontrollable voiding? Is the incontinence positional? Does it ever occur in the lying or sitting positions?

Is there difficulty initiating the stream? Is pushing or straining needed to start? Is the stream weak or interrupted? Is there postvoid dribbling? Has the patient ever been in urinary retention?

In order to document the nature and severity of urinary incontinence, a micturition diary is indispensable (Fig. 2.1).

NAME:_____   DATE:_____

TIME OF URGE TO VOID	STRENGTH OF PAIN OR URGE	TIME OF ACTUAL VOID	VOIDED VOLUME	INCONTINENCE (S, U OR W) see below	AMOUNT OF LEAKAGE (LARGE=L, MEDIUM=M, SMALL=S)
1.					
2.					
3.					
4.					
5.					
6.					
7.					
8.					
9.					
10.					
11.					
12.					
13.					
14.					
15.					
16.					
17.					

Urgency is the feeling that you have to urinate badly.

Incontinence is the loss of urine control before reaching the bathroom.
S = Stress Incontinence is wetting or leakage at times of coughing, sneezing, or with physical activity, etc.
U = Urge Incontinence is wetting or leakage because of urgency.
W = Unaware Incontinence is wetting without conscious awareness of when it happens.

Fig. 2.1. Micturition diary.

PAST MEDICAL HISTORY

The patient should be asked about neurologic conditions which are known to affect bladder and sphincteric function such as multiple sclerosis, spinal cord injury, myelodysplasia, diabetes, stroke, or Parkinson's disease. In this respect it is important to ask about double vision, muscular weakness, paralysis or poor coordination, tremor, numbness, and tingling. A history of prostate surgery, vaginal surgery, or previous surgical repair of incontinence suggests the possibility of sphincteric injury, but may also cause detrusor instability. Abdominoperineal resection of the rectum, or radical hysterectomy may be associated with neurologic injury to the bladder and sphincter. Radiation therapy may cause a small capacity bladder with low compliance.

Medications are a rare cause of urinary incontinence. Sympatholytic agents may cause stress incontinence. Sympathomimetics and tricyclic antidepressants may cause bladder outlet obstruction, urinary retention, and overflow incontinence. Parasympathomimetics may cause involuntary detrusor contractions.

PHYSICAL EXAMINATION

A focused physical examination should be performed to (1) demonstrate urinary incontinence, (2) detect associated prolapse and other pelvic conditions in women, (3) detect associated prostate conditions in men, and (4) detect neurologic abnormalities that contribute to urinary incontinence.

The nature of the incontinence should be determined by examining the patient with a full bladder as discussed in the section entitled "Eyeball Urodynamics."

The neurourologic examination begins by observing the patient's gait and demeanor as he or she first enters the office. A slight limp or lack of coordination, an abnormal speech pattern, facial asymmetry, or other abnormalities may be subtle signs of a neurologic condition. The abdomen and flanks should be examined for masses, hernias, and a distended bladder. Rectal examination will disclose the size and consistency of the prostate. The sacral dermatomes are evaluated by assessing anal sphincter tone and control, perianal sensation, and the bulbocavernosus reflex. With a finger in the rectum or the vagina, the patient is asked to squeeze as if he or she were in the middle of urinating and trying to stop. A lax or weakened anal sphincter or the inability to voluntarily contract and relax are signs of neurologic damage.

The bulbocavernosus reflex is checked by suddenly squeezing the glans penis or clitoris and feeling (or seeing) the anal sphincter and perineal muscles contract. Alternatively, the reflex may be initiated by suddenly pulling the balloon of the Foley catheter against the vesical neck. The absence of this reflex in men is almost always associated with a neurologic lesion, but the reflex is not detectable in up to 30% of otherwise normal women.[3]

In women a vaginal examination should be performed with both an empty bladder (to check the pelvic organs) and a full bladder (to check for incontinence and prolapse). With the bladder comfortably full in the lithotomy position, the patient is asked to cough or strain in an attempt to reproduce the incontinence. The degree of urethral hypermobility is assessed by the Q-tip test.[4] The Q-tip test is performed by inserting a well-lubricated sterile cotton-tipped applicator gently through the urethra into the bladder. Once in the bladder, the Q-tip is withdrawn to the point of resistance which is at the level of the vesical neck. The resting angle from the horizontal is recorded. The patient is then asked to strain and the degree of rotation is assessed. Hypermobility is defined as a resting or straining angle of greater than 30° from the horizontal and is equivalent to stress incontinence type II, provided that incontinence is demonstrated. When the findings are inconclusive, the examination should be repeated in the standing position.

The anterior vaginal wall is examined by applying gentle pressure on the posterior vaginal wall with the posterior blade from a split vaginal speculum. The blade, if metal, should be warmed with water and inserted into the vagina, depressing the posterior vaginal wall. While the patient is straining, the presence of a cystocele and cervical mobility are assessed at their full extent. Women with prolapse, including cystocele, uterine prolapse, or rectocele require careful examination in both lithotomy and sitting or standing positions. The design of our urodynamic chair and modifications of birthing chairs allows the perineum to be visualized and examined while the patient is sitting. We have found prolapse and incontinence present while the patient is sitting and not in lithotomy and vice versa. Careful reduction of the cystocele (either manually or with a pessary) in both positions may be necessary to demonstrate stress incontinence. The cervix is normally mobile, however, descent to the introitus is abnormal.

After the anterior vaginal wall has been examined, the blade is rotated and the anterior vagina gently retracted. The posterior vaginal wall and vault are examined for the presence of a rectocele or enterocele. As the speculum is slowly withdrawn, a transverse groove separating an enterocele from a rectocele below may be visible and a finger inserted in the rectum can "tent up" a rectocele but not an enterocele. An enterocele may not be detected during examination and found at the time of cystocele or rectocele repair.

If incontinence is not demonstrated in lithotomy or sitting positions, the examination is repeated in the standing position. The standing position also facilitates the diagnosis of prolapse and is particularly useful for distinguishing between an enterocele and a rectocele. The patient is positioned standing facing the examiner with one foot elevated on a short stool. An enterocele will be palpable between the forefinger (in the rectum) and the thumb (in the vagina) of the same hand. The perineal body and vaginal rectal septum are examined by palpating the septum through the vagina and rectum.

The examination is concluded by palpating the uterus and lower abdomen after the patient has voided.

URODYNAMIC EVALUATION

Urodynamic evaluation is performed to determine the precise etiology of incontinence, to evaluate detrusor function, to determine the degree of pelvic floor prolapse, and to identify urodynamic risk factors for the development of upper urinary tract deterioration. These risk factors include detrusor–external sphincter dyssynergia, low bladder wall compliance, bladder outlet obstruction, and vesicoureteral reflux.

Urodynamic technique varies from "eyeball urodynamics" to sophisticated multichannel synchronous video/pressure/flow/electromyogram studies. We believe that synchronous multichannel videourodynamics offers the most comprehensive, artifact-free means of arriving at a precise diagnosis and we perform them routinely when urodynamics are indicated. When multichannel studies are not routinely performed, they should be considered under the following circumstances:

1. when simpler diagnostic tests have been inconclusive;
2. when the patient complains of incontinence, but it cannot be demonstrated clinically;

3. in patients who have previously undergone corrective surgery for incontinence;
4. in patients who have previously undergone radical pelvic surgery, such as abdominoperineal resection of the rectum or radical hysterectomy;
5. in patients with known or suspected neurologic disorders that might interfere with bladder or sphincter function (myelodysplasia, spinal cord injury, multiple sclerosis, herniated disc, cerebrovascular accident, Parkinson's disease and the Shy-Drager syndrome).

EYEBALL URODYNAMICS

"Eyeball urodynamics" is performed with the patient in the lithotomy position immediately after uroflow. A Foley catheter is inserted and postvoid residual urine measured. A regional neurologic examination is performed as outlined above. A 60-ml catheter tip syringe is connected to the Foley catheter and its barrel removed. Water or saline is then poured in through the open end of the syringe and allowed to drip into the bladder by gravity. As the water level in the syringe falls, its meniscus represents the intravesical pressure, which can be estimated in centimeters of water above the symphysis pubis. When the water level in the syringe falls to the level of the catheter tip, it is refilled.

During bladder filling the patient is told to neither void nor try to inhibit micturition; rather he is instructed to simply report his sensations to the examiner. When he perceives the urge to void, he is asked if that is the usual feeling which he experiences when he needs to urinate.

Changes in vesical pressure are apparent as a slowing down in the rate of fall, or a rise in the level of the fluid meniscus. A rise in pressure may be caused by a detrusor contraction, an increase in abdominal pressure, or low bladder wall compliance. As soon as a rise in pressure is noted, the examiner should attempt to determine the cause. Visual inspection will usually belie abdominal straining, but in doubtful cases the abdomen should be palpated. In most instances the cause of the rise in vesical pressure will be obvious, but when in doubt, formal cystometry with rectal pressure monitoring is necessary.

Any sudden rise in pressure which is accompanied by an urge to void or by incontinence is an involuntary detrusor contraction. In some instances, the etiology of incontinence is easily discernible as the patient voids uncontrollably around the catheter during an involuntary detrusor contraction. If involuntary detrusor contractions do not occur, the bladder is filled until a normal urge to void is experienced. The bladder is left full and the catheter removed. The presence or absence of gravitational urinary loss is noted. The patient is asked to cough and bear down with gradually increasing force in order to determine the ease with which incontinence may be produced. In women, the introitus is observed for signs of cystourethrocele, rectocele, enterocele, and uterine prolapse.

Incontinence that occurs during stress is not always due to sphincter abnormalities. In some patients, the stress initiates a reflex detrusor contraction. This condition has been termed *stress hyperreflexia*. Thus, it is important to determine whether the leakage is accompanied by descent of the bladder base and urethra. It should be further noted whether the leakage stops as soon as the stress is over or does the patient actually continue to void uncontrollably. In the former case, the patient has the condition *stress incontinence;* in the latter, it is *stress hyperreflexia*. If the patient has leakage which is clearly accompanied by descent of the bladder base and proximal urethra (a cystourethrocele) and the leakage stops as soon as the cough or strain is over, she has type I or II stress incontinence. If the leakage occurs without descent, or with minimal provocation, she may have sphincteric incontinence (type III stress incontinence).[2]

If the patient complains of urinary incontinence, but it has not been demonstrated, the examination should be repeated in the standing position. It is best performed by having the patient stand with one foot on a small stool. The examiner sits beside her and performs a vaginal exam while she coughs and strains. If the examiner is still unable to demonstrate the incontinence, the patient is given a prescription for a urinary dye, such as pyridium, and asked to wear incontinence pads and tampons which she changes ever 4 h for a single representative day. She is instructed to bring the stained pads and tampons with her to the next office visit. The amount and location of the staining may help to determine the site and degree of urinary loss. It is axiomatic that, under ordinary circumstances, no patient should undergo invasive or irreversible treatment until the etiology of the incontinence has been clearly demonstrated.

LABORATORY URODYNAMICS

Laboratory urodynamics relies on the same general principles as "eyeball urodynamics," however, the measurements of pressure and flow are recorded electronically rather than visually. In addition, other physiologic parameters, such as sphincter electromyography, are not possible to evaluate without electronics. The addition of fluoroscopic evaluation of the lower urinary tract is another valuable diagnostic tool which is not possible without sophisticated equipment. The main advantage of laboratory urodynamics is the ability to record and display multiple parameters simultaneously. Not only does this provide a more precise understanding of physiology, but the individual findings serve as a check against one another to minimize the likelihood of misinterpretation of the findings. A detailed discussion of urodynamic technique is beyond the scope of this chapter. The interested reader is referred to the original references cited below.

Cystometry

From a technical standpoint, cystometry is the graphic representation of intravesical pressure as a function of bladder volume. It is used to assess detrusor activity, sensation, capacity, and compliance.[1,5] According to the International Continence Society, detrusor activity may be either normal or overactive.[1] The overactive detrusor is characterized by involuntary detrusor contractions which may be spontaneous or provoked by rapid filling, changes in position, coughing, or other triggering maneuvers. When involuntary detrusor contractions are due to neurologic disorders, the condition is called *detrusor hyperreflexia*. In the absence of a demonstrable neurologic etiology, the proper term to describe involuntary detrusor contractions is *detrusor instability*. Bladder sensation may be described as normal, absent, hypersensitive, or hyposensitive. Bladder compliance is defined as σvolume/σpressure.[1] Low compliance has been shown to be a significant risk factor for developing upper urinary tract complications.[6]

The bladder is filled at a rate which is determined by the patient's symptoms. In most instances, medium fill cystometry is appropriate (filling rates between 10–100 ml/min), but slower rates may be advisable in patients with sensory urge syndromes. The rest of the cystometric examination is performed as described above in the section on "eyeball urodynamics." The main disadvantage of "eyeball urodynamics" and one-channel cystometry is that it may be very difficult to detect the presence of detrusor contractions, particularly if they are of small magnitude. Electronic cystometry overcomes this problem because vesical, abdominal, and detrusor pressure can be measured separately. This enables the detection of detrusor contractions which might otherwise be masked by the effects of abdominal pressure on the vesical pressure tracing (Fig. 2.2).

From a clinical standpoint there is little difference whether gas or liquid is used as the infusant for cystometry.[7-10] Either results in the same clinical diagnosis. However, all of the numerical values for the volume at which events occur (such as bladder capacity) are reduced by about one-third when gas is used instead of liquid. In our opinion, liquid is far superior to gas for a number of reasons. Liquid is much more versatile. If incontinence occurs during the cystometrogram it is usually obvious. Gas leakage is much more difficult to detect. When liquid is used, the bladder can be left full at the conclusion of the study, the patient checked for stress incontinence and uroflow obtained. This is impossible with gas. In addition, liquid is more physiologic. It is not compressible like gas and it is much less irritating. Thus, the volume of fluid infused is a fairly accurate measure of the bladder volume. Finally, most gas cystometers have the capability of infusion at very high rates of flow (up to 300 ml/min). The resulting rapid fill cystometrograms often defy clinical interpretation because of the superimposition of the viscoelastic properties of the bladder wall on the physiologic properties of the bladder. In many of these studies using gas, it is almost impossible to distinguish a detrusor contraction from low bladder compliance.

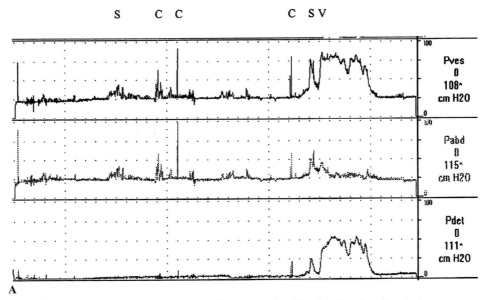

Fig. 2.2. Representative cystometrograms. The top tracing (Pves) is the plot of vesical pressure versus bladder volume and is the graph that appears as single-channel cystometry. The middle tracing (Pabd) is abdominal pressure and the lower plot is detrusor pressure (Pdet) which is electronically calculated by subtraction of Pves − Pabd. **A:** Normal increases in abdominal pressure from straining (S) and coughing (C) appear on the Pves tracing as increases in pressure which might be confused with detrusor contractions, but display of Pdet obviates this potential source of artifact. A voluntary detrusor contraction is seen at (V).

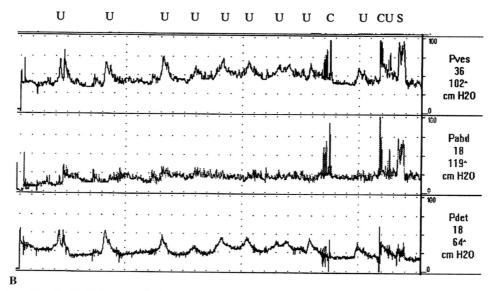

B

Fig. 2.2. B: Multiple unstable detrusor contractions (U). C = cough, S = strain.

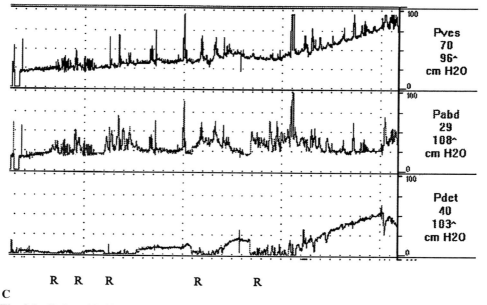

C

Fig. 2.2. C: Low bladder compliance. Low compliance is evident on the cystometric tracing (Pves) as a steep rise in pressure which reaches nearly 100 cm H_2O at a bladder capacity of 405 ml. Spontaneous rectal contractions (R) cause an artifactual decrease in detrusor pressure (Pdet).

Urinary Flow Rate

Urinary flow rate is a composite measure of the interaction between the pressure generated by the detrusor and the resistance offered by the urethra. Thus, a low uroflow may be due either to bladder outlet obstruction or impaired detrusor contractility.[11] Moreover, a normal uroflow may be seen in patients with urethral obstruction if they generate a high enough detrusor pressure to overcome the increased urethral resistance. In order to distinguish between obstruction and impaired detrusor contractility, it is necessary to measure detrusor pressure and uroflow simultaneously. Thus, a normal uroflow does not necessarily mean that the detrusor is normal, nor does it mean that the patient will be able to void after corrective surgery for incontinence. Representative uroflows are seen in Fig. 2.3.

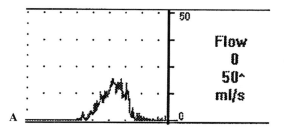

Fig. 2.3. Characteristic uroflows **A:** Normal

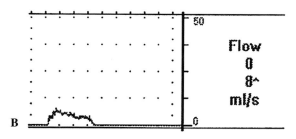

B: Prostatic obstruction

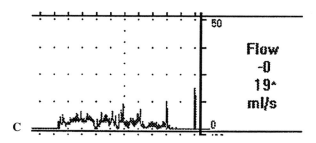

C: Impaired detrusor contractility.

Leak Point Pressure

The leak point pressure is a measure of sphincteric function. It is the lowest pressure at which urinary leakage occurs during Valsalva or cough, in the absence of a detrusor contraction. Conceptually, it is useful for two types of patients—those with stress incontinence and those with low bladder compliance. In patients with low bladder compliance, the detrusor leak point pressure is measured by filling the bladder and determining the detrusor pressure at which there is leakage from the urethra. McGuire has documented the deleterious effects that a high detrusor leak point pressure has on the upper urinary tracts; leak point pressures greater than 40 cm H_2O result in hydronephrosis or vesicoureteral reflux in 85% of myelodysplastic patients.[6]

In patients with incontinence, the vesical leak point pressure appears to be a good index of sphincteric function. The technique is as follows. The bladder is filled until the patient is either comfortably full or to a preset volume. She is asked to perform a Valsalva maneuver, progressively increasing abdominal pressure until urinary leakage is seen at the meatus or by x-ray. Vesical and abdominal pressure are measured and the leak point pressure is defined as the lowest vesical pressure that causes leakage.

Conceptually, women with low leak point pressures have intrinsic sphincter deficiency. McGuire has suggested 60 cm H_2O as a cut-off; values below that are considered to have intrinsic sphincter deficiency. The test may be grossly inaccurate in patients with significant cystocele. Patients who do not leak with Valsalva probably have a "good," intrinsic sphincter mechanism, but the effect of voluntary striated muscle control during Valsalva has not been studied well enough to determine whether or not there are false negative results.[12]

Cystogram and Voiding Cystourethrogram

Radiologic visualization of the lower urinary tract during bladder filling and voiding are useful for determining the site of bladder outlet obstruction, the integrity of the sphincter mechanism, and the presence of vesicoureteral reflux, bladder diverticula, and trabeculations of the bladder wall. Fluoroscopic monitoring during filling, voiding, and provocative maneuvers such as straining or coughing is far preferable to static films. In general, when these studies cannot be performed at the same time as urodynamic evaluation, it is better to perform the urodynamic studies first so that the functional status of the bladder and urethra are known at the time of radiologic examination. Clinical examples of voiding cystourethrograms are seen in Fig. 2.4.

Detrusor Pressure/Uroflow Studies

The simultaneous measurement of detrusor pressure and uroflow allows for the distinction between normal, urethral obstruction and impaired detrusor contractility. In fact, there is no other technique currently available to make these distinctions.[11] Urethral obstruction is defined by measuring a detrusor contraction of adequate pressure and duration in the face of a low flow. Impaired detrusor contractility is diagnosed when a low flow is accompanied by a detrusor contraction of low pressure or short duration. For a detailed discussion of techniques, interpretation, and computer analysis, the reader is referred to several reviews.[5,13–17] Pressure flow studies are performed at the conclusion of the cystometrogram. The patient voids and detrusor pressure is measured with a small urethral (4–10 Fr)

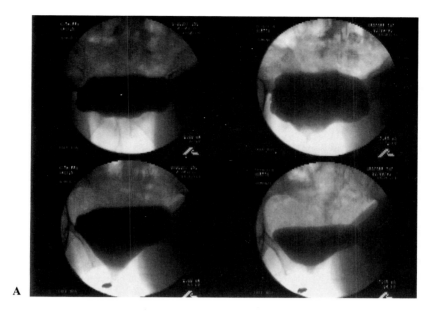

Fig. 2.4. Representative voiding cystourethrograms. By simply viewing these films, there is no way of determining the functional significance. Are these patients voiding normally or is there incontinence? Is there urethral obstruction? Only by verbal interaction with the patient and measurement of urodynamic parameters can the diagnosis be appreciated.
A: Selected films from a woman voiding normally.

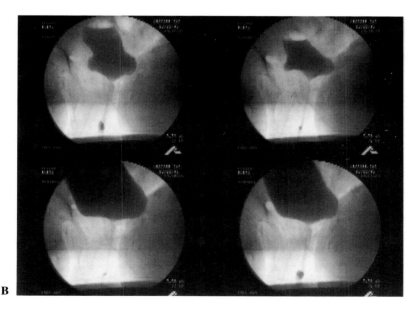

B: Selected films from a man with detrusor hyperreflexia and prostatic obstruction.

or suprapubic catherter while uroflow is simultaneously measured. Representative pressure flow studies are depicted in Fig. 2.5.

Sphincter Electromyography

Electromyography is only rarely indicated for the evaluation of urinary incontinence. For practical purposes, the only instance in which it is necessary is when there is suspicion of a neurologic lesion which requires more objective documentation, or when a bonafide neurologic lesion requires further characterization. Sphincter electromyography plays a dual role. In an indirect way it provides kinesiologic information about the urethral sphincter and the pelvic floor muscles. It also provides objective data about the integrity of the innervation to these muscles and the synchronization between detrusor and external sphincter. In order to objectively evaluate innervation, the electromyogram (EMG) must be performed by an experienced examiner using needle electrodes and oscilloscopic or audio control.[5]

Urethral Pressure Profilometry

Despite an abundant literature on urethral profilometry, it is our opinion that routine measurement of urethral pressures is neither necessary nor useful in the evaluation of incontinence.[18] A number of new techniques have been described which measure pressure transmission ratios from bladder to urethra during increases in intra-abdominal pressure, but their clinical applicability has yet to be proven. The micturitional static urethral pressure

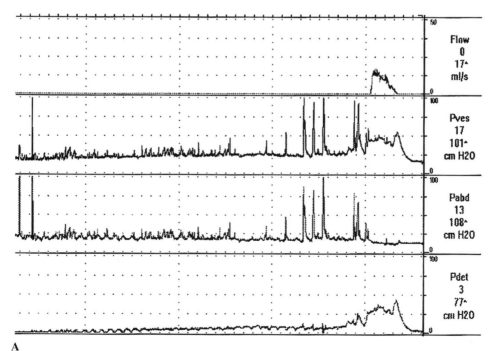

A

Fig. 2.5. Detrusor pressure/uroflow studies.
A: Normal.

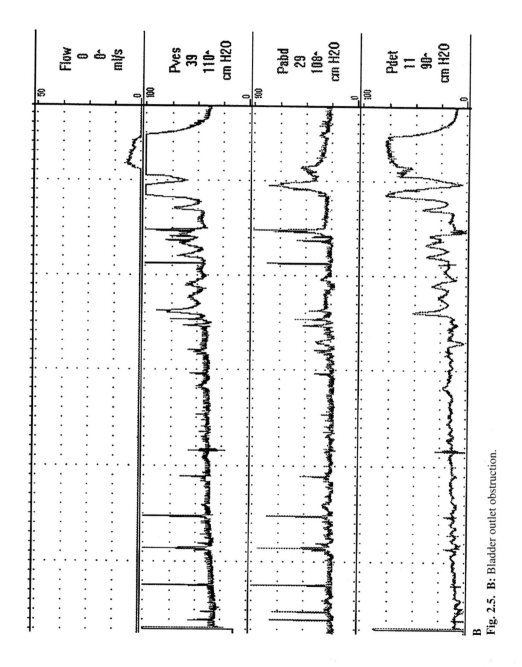

Fig. 2.5. B: Bladder outlet obstruction.

B

37

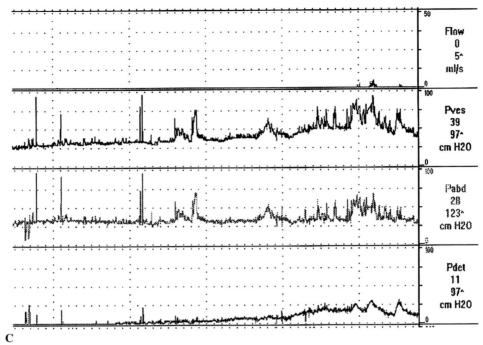

C

Fig. 2.5. C: Impaired detrusor contractility.

profile as described by Yalla et al.[19,20] is a useful means of diagnosing the site of urethral obstruction, but is not necessary for routine evaluation.

Videourodynamics

Synchronous measurement and display of urodynamic parameters with radiographic visualization of the lower urinary tract videourodynamics is the most precise diagnostic tool for evaluating disturbances of micturition.[5] In these studies, radiographic contrast is used as the infusant for cystometry. Depending on the level of sophistication required, other urodynamic parameters such as abdominal pressure, urethral pressure, uroflow, and sphincter electromyography may be recorded as well. There are important advantages to synchronous video/pressure flow studies compared to conventional single-channel urodynamics and to conventional cystography and voiding cystourethrography. By simultaneously measuring multiple urodynamic variables one gains a better insight into the underlying pathophysiology. Moreover, since all variables are visualized simultaneously one can better appreciate their interrelationships and identify artifacts with ease. Representative videourodynamic studies are depicted in Fig. 2.6.

TREATMENT OVERVIEW

Treatment of incontinence should be predicated on a clear understanding of the underlying physiology.

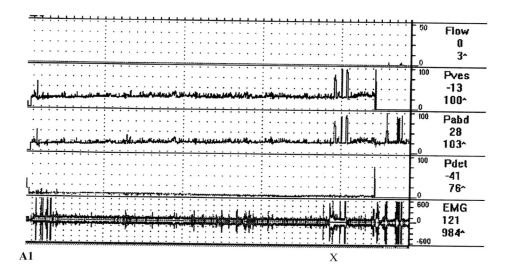

A1   X

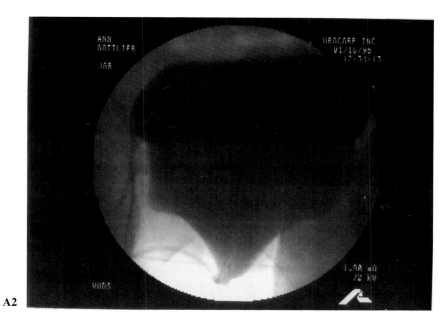

A2

Fig. 2.6. Representative videourodynamic studies. **A1 & A2:** Type II stress incontinence. The x-ray was exposed at point X at a leak point pressure $=100$ cm H_2O.

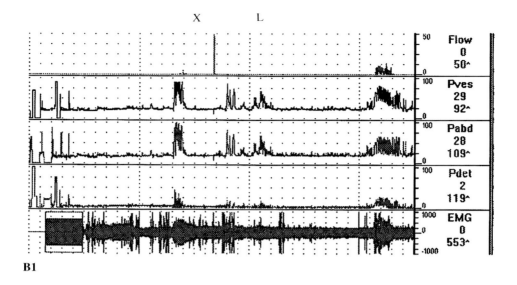

B1

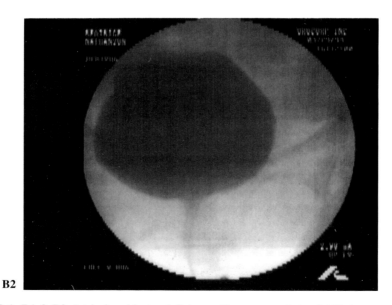

B2

Fig. 2.6. B1 & B2: Intrinsic sphincter deficiency. X-ray exposed at point X shows an open vesical neck at rest. Leak point pressure was 37 cm H$_2$O (L).

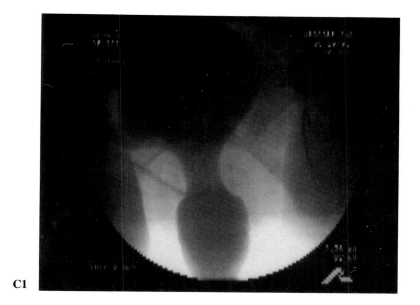

C1

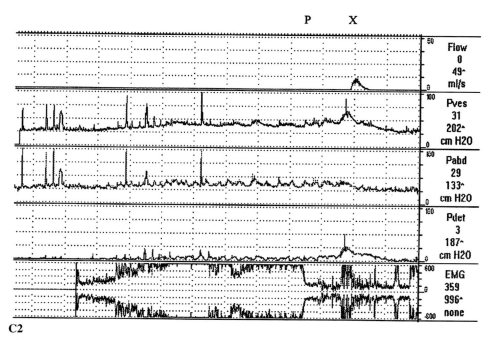

C2

Fig. 2.6. C1 & C2: Detrusor instability and grade 4 cystocele. Sixty-seven-year-old white woman with a chief complaint of "dropped bladder" and urge incontinence. X-ray exposed at P shows a grade 4 cystocele and at X she voided with an unstable detrusor contraction to 25 cm H_2O.

Detrusor Instability (Involuntary Detrusor Contractions)

The ideal approach to the treatment of urinary incontinence due to involuntary detrusor contractions is to eliminate the underlying etiology. Although this is rarely possible when the cause is neurologic or idiopathic, in patients with urethral obstruction, the symptoms of detrusor instability are ameliorated in the majority of patients after the obstruction has been cured. Urethral obstruction is rare in women and usually caused by previous pelvic surgery. In men, urethral obstruction is usually due to benign prostatic hyperplasia (BPH) and symptomatic relief of detrusor instability is expected in over two-thirds of men who undergo successful transurethral resection of the prostate (TURP).

When it is not possible to treat the underlying etiology, the basic treatment is to abolish the involuntary detrusor contractions. This may be accomplished by a variety of therapeutic modalities including medications (anticholinergics, musculotropic relaxing agents, and tricyclic antidepressants) behavior modification, electrical stimulation, and biofeedback. In refractory patients with detrusor instability, augmentation enterocystoplasty is effective in the great majority of patients, but many will require intermittent self-catheterization.

A detailed discussion of these treatment modalities is presented in subsequent chapters.

Stress Urinary Incontinence

In general, surgical treatment of stress incontinence is far more successful than nonsurgical treatment. Medications (α-adrenergic agonists), biofeedback, electrical stimulation, and behavior modification have all been reported to cause improvement in 30–75% of patients but cure is usually not possible with these therapeutic modalities. These treatments are discussed in detail in succeeding chapters.

Selection of the type of surgery is based primarily on the underlying anatomic and physiologic abnormalities responsible for incontinence. There are five generic kinds of procedures for stress incontinence: periurethral injection, transvaginal vesical neck suspension, retropubic urethropexy, pubovaginal sling, and sphincter prosthesis. Each of these is discussed in detail in later chapters. An overview of surgical treatment based on the underlying pathophysiology is presented below.

Urethral Hypermobility (Stress Incontinence Type II A and B)

The basic principle of surgical treatment or urethral hypermobility is to prevent the abnormal descent of the urethra which occurs during increases in intra-abdominal pressure. This may be accomplished with any of the standard urethropexy operations, such as the Marshall-Marchetti-Krantz or Burch, the needle bladder neck suspension procedures (modified Peyrera procedure), or creation of a pubovaginal sling. The role of periurethral injection of collagen, autologous fat, polytef, and other implantable substances is currently under investigation, but preliminary data suggests that the injectables have an unacceptably low success rate in patients with hypermobility.

In some women, particularly those who have undergone previous pelvic surgery, there is scarring and fixation of the vesical neck and proximal urethra to the anterior vaginal wall. In these patients, surgical treatment is designed to restore these structures to their normal anatomic position by freeing them of their vaginal attachments, then preventing abnormal descent by any of the above procedures.

Intrinsic Sphincter Deficiency (Stress Incontinence Type III)

In Type III SUI, the proximal urethra no longer functions as a sphincter. Since the problem is not one of abnormal descent, the usual suspension operations for SUI are often unsuccessful. A sphincter prosthesis is theoretically ideal, but has an unacceptably high failure rate in patients who have had multiple prior surgeries. In these patients a pubovaginal sling has the operation of choice. The periurethral injection of collagen, autologous fat, polytef, and other implantable substances shows great promise. The short-term efficacy in women has been documented, but long-term studies have not been done and it is not known how often these injections must be repeated.

Type O and I Stress Incontinence

In Type O and I stress incontinence, the relative contributions of hypermobility and intrinsic sphincter deficiency (ISD) may be difficult to assess. An estimation of the pressure necessary to induce incontinence such as the abdominal leak point pressure is the most useful diagnostic technique currently available to make this distinction. We believe that patients with Type I SUI are a forme fruste of ISD and appear to respond well to periurethral injections.

Stress Incontinence Associated with Urethral Diverticulum

The preoperative evaluation of patients with urethral diverticulum should include a careful assessment for stress urinary incontinence. When both are present, they should be repaired at the same time adhering to the principles outlined above. It should be recognized that during the vaginal dissection the vesical neck supports may become weakened and an iatrogenic stress incontinence may ensue. To prevent this the surgeon should consider making an intraoperative decision to correct the potential anatomic condition whenever necessary.

Stress Incontinence Associated with Vesicovaginal or Urethrovaginal Fistula

Whenever there is urinary incontinence associated with a vesicovaginal or urethrovaginal fistula, a careful evaluation should be undertaken to ensure that the patient does not have sphincteric incontinence in addition to the fistula. If sphincteric incontinence is documented, it should be repaired at the same time as the fistula repair.

Mixed Incontinence (Incontinence due to Sphincter Abnormalities and Detrusor Instability)

Approximately 30–50% of women with stress incontinence also complain of urinary frequency, urgency, and/or urge incontinence. In addition to the routine workup, these patients should have careful evaluation including urinary cytology and cystourethroscopy. Conditions such as carcinoma in situ of the bladder, bladder stones, and interstitial cystitis should be excluded. When the stress symptoms predominate, and stress incontinence is objectively demonstrated, surgical repair will usually alleviate all of their symptoms. However, when the other symptoms predominate, or when the degree of stress incontinence seems minimal compared to the severity of the urge symptoms, repair of the stress incontinence may not be helpful at all, and may even intensify the patient's complaints. Whenever there is doubt, it is most reasonable to proceed with noninvasive medical treatment of the frequency/urgency symptoms prior to consideration of surgical therapy of stress incontinence.

POSTPROSTATECTOMY INCONTINENCE

The vast majority of postprostatectomy sphincteric incontinence subsides spontaneously in the first few weeks to months after surgery. For persistent incontinence, conservative therapies such as α-adrenergic agonists, biofeedback, electrical stimulation, and behavior modification should be tried, but for incontinence that persists longer than a year after surgery surgical treatment is generally the only reasonable long-term solution unless the patient prefers to manage the problem with absorbent pads, condom catheters, a penile clamp, or an indwelling catheter.

The most successful surgical treatment is the implantation of a sphincter prosthesis with a reported success rate of 80–90%. The role of periurethral injections is still under investigation but to date has been disappointing with short-term cure rates of no more than 15%. In general, periurethral injections appear to be more successful in patients with post-TURP incontinence than after radical prostatectomy. A detailed discussion of these treatments is presented in Chapter 8.

REFERENCES

1. Abrams P, Blaivas JG, Stanton SL, et al: Standardisation of lower urinary tract function. *Neurourol Urodyn* 7:403, 1988.

2. Blaivas JG, Olsson CA: Stress incontinence: classification and surgical approach. *J Urol* 139:737, 1988.

3. Blaivas JG: The bulbocavernosus reflex in urology: a prospective study of 299 patients. *J Urol* 126:197, 1981.

4. Wall LL, Norton PA, DeLancey JOL: Prolapse and the lower urinary tract. In Wall LL, Norton PA, DeLancey JOL (eds): *Practical Urogynecology.* Baltimore, 1993, pp 293–315.

5. Blaivas JG: Techniques of evaluation. Yalla SV, McGuire EJ, Elbadawi A, et al(eds): *Neurourology and Urodynamics, Principles and Practice.* New York, Macmillan, 1988.

6. McGuire EJ, Woodside JR, Borden TA, et al: The prognostic significance of urodynamic testing in myelodysplastic patients. *J Urol* 125:205, 1981.

7. Cass AS, Ward BD, Markland C: Comparison of slow and rapid fill cystometry using liquid and air. *J Urol* 104:104, 1970.

8. Gleason DM, Bottaccini MR, Reilly RJ: Comparison of cystometrograms and urethral Iprofiles with gas and water media. *Urology* 9:155, 1977.

9. Jorgensen L, Lose G, Andersen JT: Cystometry: H_2O and CO_2 as the filling medium? A literature survey of the influence of the filling media on the qualitative and the quantitative cystometric parameters. *Neurourol Urodyn* 7:343, 1988.

10. Merrill DC, Bradley WE, Markland C: Air cystometry. II. A clinical evaluation of normal adults. *J Urol* 108:85, 1972.

11. Chancellor MB, Blaivas JG, Kaplan SA, et al: Bladder outlet obstruction versus impaired detrusor contractility: role of uroflow. *J Urol* 145:810, 1991.

12. McGuire EJ, Fitzpatrick CC, Wan J, et al: Clinical assessment of urethral sphincter function. *J Urol* 150:1452, 1993.

13. Griffiths DJ: *Urodynamics: The Mechanics of Hydrodynamics of the Lower Urinary Tract.* Medical Physics Handbooks, vol 4. Bristol, England, Hilger, 1980.

14. Griffiths DJ: The mechanics of micturition. In Yalla SV, Elbadawi A, McGuire E, et al: *The Principles and Practice of Neurourology and Urodynamics.* New York, Macmillan, 1988.

15. Schafer W: Urethral resistance? Urodynamic concepts of physiological and pathological bladder outlet function during voiding. *Neurourol Urodyn* 4:161, 1985.

16. Schafer W: Detrusor as the energy source of micturition. In Hinman F Jr (ed): *Benign Prostatic Hypertrophy.* New York, Springer-Verlag, 1983.

17. Schafer W, Waterbar F, Langen PH, et al: A simplified graphical procedure for detailed analysis of detrusor and outlet function during voiding, *Neurourol Urodyn* 8:405, 1989.

18. Blaivas JG, Awad SA, Bissada N, et al: Urodynamic procedure: recommendations of the Urodynamic Society 1. Procedures that should be available for routine urologic practice. *Neurourol Urodyn* 1:51, 1982.

19. Yalla SV, Sharma GVRK, Barsamian EM: Micturitional urethral pressure profile during voiding and the implications. *J Urol* 124:629, 1980.

20. Yalla SV, Bute R, Waters W, et al: Urodynamic evaluation of prostatic enlargements with micturitional vesicourethal static pressure profiles. *J Urol* 125:684, 1981.

3

Pharmacologic Therapy of Urinary Incontinence

Alan J. Wein
Denise A. Nigro

The lower urinary tract performs two basic functions: the storage and emptying of urine. Despite disagreements on various details, all experts would doubtless agree that, for the purposes of description and teaching, one can succinctly summarize the two phases of micturition from a conceptual point of view. Bladder filling and urine storage require:

1. Accommodation of increasing volume of urine at a low intravesical pressure and with appropriate sensation.
2. A bladder outlet which is closed at rest and remains so during increases in intra-abdominal pressure.
3. Absence of involuntary bladder contractions (detrusor instability or hyperreflexia).

Bladder emptying requires:

1. A coordinated contraction of adequate magnitude and duration by the bladder smooth musculature.
2. Concomitant lowering of resistance at the level of the smooth sphincter (the smooth muscle of the bladder neck and proximal urethra) and of the striated sphincter (the periurethral and intramural urethral striated musculature).
3. Absence of anatomic obstruction.

This simple overview implies that any type of voiding dysfunction (i.e., of storage, of emptying, or a combination) must result from an abnormality of one or more of the factors listed above. This description, with its implied subdivisions under each category, provides a logical framework for the discussion and classification of all types of voiding dysfunction. In addition, all aspects of urodynamic, radiologic, and videourodynamic evaluation can be conceptualized as to exactly what they evaluate in terms of either bladder or outlet activity during filling/storage or emptying, and whether they do so by an

TABLE 3.1. Therapy to Facilitate Bladder Filling and Urine Storage

INHIBITING BLADDER CONTRACTILITY/DECREASING SENSORY INPUT/INCREASING BLADDER CAPACITY

1. Behavioral therapy
   a. Timed bladder emptying
   b. Bladder training; biofeedback
2. Pharmacologic therapy
   a. Anticholinergic agents
   b. Musculotropic relaxants
   c. Calcium antagonists
   d. Postassium channel openers
   e. Prostaglandin inhibitors
   f. β-Adrenergic agonists
   g. α-Adrenergic antagonists
   h. Tricyclic antidepressants
   i. Dimethyl sulfoxide (DMSO)
   j. Polysynaptic inhibitors
   k. Decreasing sensory input
3. Bladder overdistention
4. Electrical stimulation (reflex inhibition)
5. Acupuncture
6. Interruption of innervation
   a. Central (subarachnoid block)
   b. Sacral rhizotomy, selective sacral rhizotomy
   c. Perivesical (peripheral bladder denervation)
7. Augmentation cystoplasty

action that is primarily on the bladder, or on one or more of the components of the bladder outlet.

As a result of advances in knowledge of the neuropharmacology and neurophysiology of the lower urinary tract, pharmacologic therapy does exist that is effective in the management of many types of voiding dysfunction. This chapter will summarize those treatments available for urinary incontinence (storage failure) within this functional classification. (Table 3.1). As an apology to others in the field whose works have not been specifically cited in this chapter, it should be noted that the citations have generally been chosen primarily because of their review or informational content and not because of originality or initial publication on a particular subject.

THERAPY TO FACILITATE URINARY STORAGE/BLADDER FILLING

Decreasing Bladder Contractility/Decreasing Sensory Input

Anticholinergic Agents: General Discussion

The major portion of the neurohumoral stimulus for physiologic bladder contraction is acetylcholine (ACh)-induced stimulation of postganglionic parasympathetic muscarinic cholinergic receptor sites on bladder smooth muscle. Atropine and atropine-like agents will therefore depress normal bladder contractions and involuntary bladder contractions (IBC) of any etiology.[1] In such patients the volume at which the first IBC occurs will generally be increased, the amplitude of the IBC decreased, and the bladder capacity increased.[2-4] However, although the volume and pressure threshold at which an IBC is elicited may increase, the "warning time" (the time between the perception of an IBC about to occur and its occurrence) and the ability to suppress it are not increased. Thus, urgency and incontinence will still occur unless such therapy is combined with a regimen of timed voiding or toileting. The effect of anticholinergics in those patients who exhibit only decreased compliance has not been well studied. Outlet resistance, at least as reflected by urethral pressure measurements, does not seem to be clinically affected.

Anticholinergic Agents—Specific Drugs

Propantheline bromide (Probanthine, others). This is the classically described oral agent for producing an antimuscarinic effect in the lower urinary tract. The usual adult oral dosage is 15 to 30 mg every 4–6 hr, although higher doses are often necessary. Propantheline is a quaternary ammonium compound, all of which are poorly absorbed after oral administration.[5] There seems to be little difference between the antimuscarinic effects of propantheline on bladder smooth muscle and those of other antimuscarinic agents. There is relatively little evaluable data on the effectiveness of propantheline for the treatment of bladder hyperactivity. There are reports of both great and poor efficacy. The Agency for Health Care Policy and Research (AHCPR) clinical practice guidelines[6] list five randomized controlled trials reviewed for propantheline, with 82% female patients. Percent cures (all figures refer to percent effect on drug *minus* percent effect on placebo) are listed as 0 to 5%, reduction in urge incontinence as 0 to 53%, and percent side effects and percent dropouts as 0 to 50% and 0 to 9% respectively.

Hyoscyamine (Cystospaz) and *hyoscyamine sulfate* (Levsin/Levsinex, Cystospaz-M) are reported to have about the same general anticholinergic actions and side effects as the other belladonna alkaloids. Hyoscyamine sulfate is available as a sublingual formulation (Levsin SL)—a theoretical advantage—but controlled studies of its effects on bladder hyperactivity are lacking. *Glycopyrrolate* (Robinul) is a synthetic quaternary ammonium compound which is a potent inhibitor of both M_1 and M_2 receptors but with a preference for the M_2 subtype.[7] It is available as both an oral and parenteral preparation; the latter is commonly used as an antisialogue during anesthesia.

All antimuscarinic compounds tend to affect parasympathetically innervated organs in the same order, with generally larger doses required to inhibit bladder activity than to affect salivary, bronchial, nasopharyngeal, and sweat secretions. The potential effects of all antimuscarinic agents include inhibition of salivary secretion (dry mouth), blockade of the ciliary muscle of the lens to cholinergic stimulation (blurred vision for near objects), tachycardia, drowsiness, and inhibition of gut motility. Those agents that possess some ganglionic blocking activity may also cause orthostatic hypotension and impotence at high doses (generally required for the nicotinic activity to manifest itself). Antimuscarinic agents are generally contraindicated in patients with narrow angle glaucoma and should be used with caution in patients with significant bladder outlet obstruction, as complete urinary retention may be precipitated.

Musculotropic Relaxants

These agents fall under the general heading of direct-acting smooth muscle depressants, whose antispasmodic activity reportedly is directly on smooth muscle at a site that is metabolically distal to the cholinergic or other contractile receptor mechanism. Although all of the agents to be discussed do relax smooth muscle in vitro by papaverine-like (direct) activity, all have been found to possess variable anticholinergic and local anesthetic properties in addition. There is still a significant question as to how much of their clinical efficacy is due only to their atropine-like effect. If in fact any of these agents do exert a clinically significant inhibitory effect that is independent of antimuscarinic action, there exists a therapeutic rationale for combining their use with that of a relatively pure anticholinergic agent.

Oxybutynion chloride (Ditropan) is a moderately potent anticholinergic agent with a strong independent musculotropic relaxant activity, and local anesthetic activity as well. Comparatively higher concentrations in vitro are necessary for the direct spasmolytic effects, which may be due to calcium channel blockade.[8,9] The recommended oral adult dose is 5 mg three times a day (TID) or four times a day (QID); the side effects are antimuscarinic and dose-related. Initial reports documented success in depressing detrusor hyperreflexia in patients with neurogenic bladder dysfunction;[10] subsequent reports documented success in inhibiting other types of bladder hyperactivity as well.[11] A randomized, double-blind, placebo-controlled study comparing 5 mg oxybutynin TID with placebo in 30 patients with detrusor instability was carried out by Moisey et al.[12] Seventeen of 23 patients who completed the study with oxybutynin had a symptomatic improvement, and nine had evidence of urodynamic improvement—mainly an increase in maximal bladder capacity. Hehir and Fitzpatrick[13] found 16 of 24 patients with neuropathic voiding dysfunction secondary to myelomeningocele were cured or improved (17% dry, 50% improved) with oxybutynin treatment. Average bladder capacity increased from 197 ml to 299 (drug) versus 218 ml (placebo). Maximum bladder filling pressure decreased from 47 cm H_2O to 37 (drug) versus 45 cm H_2O (placebo). In a prospective randomized study of 34 patients with voiding dysfunction secondary to multiple sclerosis, Gajewski and Awad[14] found that 5 mg TID of oral oxybutynin produced a good response more frequently than 15 mg of propantheline TID.

Holmes et al.[15] compared the results of oxybutynin and propantheline in a small group of women with detrusor instability. The experimental design was a randomized crossover trial with a patient-regulated, variable-dose regimen. This concept of a dose titration study allows the patient to increase the drug dose to what he/she perceives to be the optimum ratio, if any, between clinical improvement and side effects—an interesting way of comparing two drugs while minimizing differences in oral absorption. Of the 23 women in the trial, 14 reported subjective improvement with oxybutynin, 11 with propantheline. Both drugs significantly increased the maximum cystometric capacity and reduced the maximum detrusor pressure on filling. The only significant objective difference was a greater increase in the maximum cystometric capacity with oxybutynin. The mean total daily dose of oxybutynin tolerated was 15 mg (range 7.5–30) and that of propantheline was 90 mg (45–145).

Thuroff et al.[16] compared oxybutynin versus propantheline versus placebo in a group of patients with symptoms of instability and either detrusor instability or hyperreflexia. Oxybutunin (5 mg TID) performed best, but propantheline was used at a relatively low dose—

15 mg TID. The rate of side effects was higher for oxybutynin at just about the level of the clinical and urodynamic improvement. Mean grade of improvement on a visual analogue scale was higher for oxybutynin (58.2%) versus propantheline (44.7%) and placebo (43.4%). The urodynamic volume at the first IBC was increased more with oxybutynin (51 ml versus 11.2 versus −9.7), as was the change in maximum cystometric capacity (80.1 ml versus 48.9 versus 22.5). Residual urine volume was also increased more (27.0 ml versus −2.2 versus −1.9). The authors further subdivided their overall results into excellent (>75% improvement), good (50–74%), fair (25–49%), and poor (<25%). Their oxybutynin percentages were, respectively, 42%, 25%, 15%, and 18%. They compared their 67% rate of good/excellent results to seven other oxybutynin series in the literature (some admittedly poorer studies included) and concluded that this compared favorably with the range of such results that they calculated from these studies (61–86%). The results of propantheline treatment were generally between those of oxybutynin and placebo, but did not reach significant levels over placebo in any variable. Similar subdivision of propantheline results yielded percentages (see above) of 20, 30, 14, and 36. The authors compared their 50% ratio of good/excellent results in five other propantheline studies in the literature (30–57%) and concluded that their results were consistent with these. Although this study is better than most in the literature, it does have drawbacks, and anyone using this in a meta-analysis would be well advised to read it and the other cited studies very carefully.

There are some negative reports on the efficacy of oxybutynin. Zorzitto et al.[17] in a double-blind, placebo-controlled trial in 24 incontinent geriatric institutionalized patients, concluded that oxybutynin 5 mg twice a day (BID) was no more effective than placebo with scheduled toileting in treating incontinence in this type of population with detrusor hyperactivity. An incontinence profile was used to assess results. The only significant difference was an increase in residual urine volume (152 versus 92 ml). Ouslander et al.[18] reported similar conclusions in a smaller study on geriatric patients, and in an accompanying article[19] concludes simply that the drug is safe for use in the elderly at doses of 2.5–5 mg three times a day. The AHCPR guideline[6] lists six randomized controlled trials for oxybutynin; 90% of patients were female. Percent cures (all figures refer to percent effect on drug *minus* percent effect on placebo) are listed as 28% and 44%, percent reduction in urge incontinence as 9–56%, and percent side effects and percent dropouts as 2–66% and 3–45% respectively.

Topical application of oxybutynin and other agents to normal or intestinal bladders has been suggested and implemented.[20] The conceptually attractive form of alternative drug delivery, either by periodic intravesical instillation of liquid or timed release pellets, awaits further clinical trials and the development of preparations specifically formulated for that purpose. Madersbacher and Jilg[21] reviewed such usage with oxybutynin and presented data on 13 patients with complete suprasacral cord lesions on clean intermittent catheterization (CIC). One 5-mg tablet was dissolved in 30 ml of distilled water and the solution instilled intravesically. Of the ten patients who were incontinent, nine remained dry for 6 hr. For the group the changes in bladder capacity and maximal detrusor pressure were statistically significant. Some of the more interesting data were in a figure which shows plasma oxybutynin levels in a group of patients in whom administration was intravesical or oral. The level following an oral dose rose to 7.3 Ng/ml within 2 hr and then precipitously dropped to slightly less than 2 Ng/ml at 4 hr. Following intravesical administration, the level rose gradually to a peak of about 6.2 at 3.5 hr, but the level at 6 hr was still greater than 4 and at 9 hr was still between 3 to 4. Did the intravesically applied drug act locally or systemically? Weese et al.[22] reported on treatment with a similar dose or oxybutynin (5 mg in 30 ml sterile water) of 42 patients with intraventricular catheter who had either failed oral anticholinergic therapy (11) or had intolerable side effects (31). Twenty had hyperreflexia, 19 instability, 3 had bowel/bladder hyperactivity after augmentation. The drug was instilled BID/TID for 10 min by catheterization. Twenty-one percent (nine patients) dropped out because of inability to tolerate CIC or retain the solution properly, but there were no reported side effects. Fifty-five percent (18/33) of patients who were able to follow the protocol reported at least a moderate subjective improvement in incontinence and urgency. Nine patients became totally continent and experienced complete resolution of their symptoms; 18 improved patients experienced a decrease of 2.5 pads per day. There were no urodynamic data. Follow-up was 5–35 months (mean 18.4). The lack of side effects prompted some speculation about the mechanism. One possibility suggested was simply a more prolonged rate of absorption. Another more intriguing one was a decreased pass through the liver and therefore a decrease in metabolites, with the hypothesis that perhaps the metabolites and not the primary compound are responsible for the side effects.

Dicyclomine hydrochloride (Bentyl) is also reported to possess a direct relaxant effect on smooth muscle in addition to an antimuscarinic action. An oral dose of 20 mg TID in adults was reported to increase bladder capacity in patients with detrusor hyperreflexia.[23] Beck et al.[24] compared the use of 10 mg dicyclomine, 15 mg propantheline, and placebo TID in patients with detrusor hyperactivity. The cure or improved rates, respectively, were 62%, 73%, and 20%. Awad et al.[25] reported that 20 mg of dicyclomine TID caused resolution or significant improvement in 24 of 27 patients with IBC.

Flavoxate hydrochloride (Urispas) is a compound that has a direct inhibitory action on smooth muscle but very weak anticholinergic properties.[11] Overall favorable clinical effects have been noted in some series of patients with frequency, urgency, and incontinence, and in patients with urodynamically documented detrusor hyperreflexia.[26] However, Briggs et al.[27] reported essentially no effect on detrusor hyperreflexia in an elderly population. A similar conclusion was reached by Chapple et al.[28] in a double-blind, placebo-controlled crossover study of the treatment of idiopathic detrusor instability with flavoxate. The recommended adult dosage is 100 to 200 mg TID or QID. As with all agents in this group, a short clinical trial may be worthwhile. Reported side effects are few.

Calcium Antagonists

The role of calcium (Ca) is well established in excitation–contraction coupling in striated, cardiac, and smooth muscle. The dependence of contractile activity on changes in cytosolic Ca varies from tissue to tissue, as do the characteristics of the Ca channels involved, but interference with Ca inflow or intracellular release is a very potent potential mechanism for bladder smooth muscle relaxation. Many experimental studies have confirmed the inhibitory effects of Ca antagonists on a variety of experimental models of spontaneous and induced-bladder muscle strip and whole bladder preparation activity, these results supporting the view that combined muscarinic receptor and Ca channel blockage might offer a more effective way of treating bladder hyperactivity than single mechanism therapies presently available. *Terodiline* is an agent with both Ca antagonist and anticholinergic properties. At low concentrations it has mainly an anticholinergic effect, whereas at higher concentrations a Ca antagonistic effect becomes evident. There have been a number of clinical studies on the inhibitory action of this compound on bladder hyperactivity, which have shown clinical effectiveness.[29] Peters et al.[30] reported the results of a multicenter study which ultimately included data from 89 patients (of an original 128) comparing terodiline and placebo in women with motor urge incontinence. The daily dose in this study was 12.5 mg in the morning and 25 mg at night. They concluded that terodiline was more effective than placebo, but noted that this improvement was much more apparent on subjective assessment than an objective assessment of cystometric and micturition data. Sixty-three percent of patients preferred terodiline, regardless of treatment sequence. Although statistically significant objective results were recorded between terodiline and placebo, these were not very impressive. Tapp et al.[31] reported on a double-blind placebo study, using a dose titration technique, which included 70 women with urodynamically proven detrusor instability and bladder capacities of less than 400 cc. Sixty-two percent of the 34 women in the terodiline group considered themselves improved, 38% unchanged. Of the 36 women in the placebo group, 42% considered themselves improved, 47% unchanged, and 11% worse, a statistically significant response in favor of the terodiline group with regard to the improvement percentage. Micturition variables of daytime frequency, daytime incontinence episodes, number of pads used, and average voided volumes were statistically changed in favor of terodiline, but the absolute changes were relatively small. Urodynamic data, while showing a trend in favor of terodiline in each parameter, showed no statistically significant differences in any category. Side effects were noted in a large number and with equal frequency in both groups after the dose titration phase. However, the incidence of anticholinergic side effects was higher in the drug group. The AHCPR guideline[6] lists seven randomized controlled risks for terodiline; 94% of patients were female. Percent cures (all figures refer to percent drug effect *minus* percent effect on placebo) are listed at 18% and 33%, percent reduction in urge incontinence as 14–83%, and percent side effects and percent dropouts as 14–40% and 2–8% respectively.

Terodiline is almost completely absorbed from the GI tract and has a low serum clearance. The recommended dosage in adults is 25 mg BID, reduced to an initial dose of 12 mg BID in geriatric patients. The half-life is around 60 hr and Abrams[29] logically proposes, on this basis, a once-daily dose, but emphasizes the necessity of dose titration for each patient. The common side effects seen with calcium antagonists (hypotension, facial flushing, headache, dizziness, abdominal discomfort, constipation, nausea, rash, weakness and palpitations) had not been reported in the larger initial clinical studies with terodilene, side effects consisting primarily of those consequent to its anticholinergic action. However, questions were raised about the occurrence of a rare arrhythmia (torsade de pointes) in patients taking terodiline simultaneously with antidepressants or antiarrhythmic drugs.[32] After further reports of apparent cardiac toxicity, the drug was voluntarily withdrawn by the manufacturer pending the results of further safety studies. The United States studies for FDA approval were likewise voluntarily halted by the manufacturer; there is currently activity directed toward their reinstitution. The problems were unfortunate, because the drug seemed quite effective and offered the additional advantages of a long half-life and the ability to titrate the dose for each patient, sometimes to a once-daily administration. Other Ca antagonist drugs have not been widely used to treat voiding dysfunction.

Potassium Channel Openers

Potassium (K) channel openers efficiently relax various types of smooth muscle by increasing K efflux, resulting in membrane hyperpolarization. Hyperpolarization reduces the opening probability of ion channels involved in membrane depolarization, and excitation is reduced.[33] There are some suggestions that bladder instability, at least that associated with infravesical obstruction and detrusor hypertrophy, might be secondary to supersensitivity to depolarizing stimuli. Theoretically, then, K channel openers might be an attractive alternative for the treatment of detrusor instability in such circumstances, without inhibiting the normal voluntary contraction necessary for bladder emptying.[34] Pinacidil is such a compound. Unfortunately, a preliminary study with this agent in a double-blind crossover format showed no effect on symptom status in nine patients with detrusor instability and bladder outlet obstruction.[35] Nurse et al.[36] reported on the use of cromkalim, another potassium channel opener, in 17 patients with refractory detrusor instability or hyperreflexia or who had stopped other drug therapy because of intolerable side effects. Six of 16 (35%) patients who completed the study showed a decrease in frequency and an increase in voided volume. Long-term observation was not possible since the drug was withdrawn because of reported adverse effects of high doses in animal toxicologic studies. Potassium channel openers are not at present very specific for bladder. If tissue-selective K activator drugs could be developed, they could prove very useful for the treatment of detrusor instability. The side effects of pinacidil have been best studied and include headache, peripheral edema (25–50% and dose-related), weight gain, palpitations, dizziness, and rhinitis. Hypertrichosis and asymptomatic T-wave changes are also reported (30%).

Prostaglandin Inhibitors

There exist multiple mechanisms whereby prostaglandin synthesis inhibitors might decrease bladder contractility in response to various stimuli. However, objective evidence that this occurs clinically is scant.

β-Adrenergic Agonists

The presence of β-adrenergic receptors in human bladder muscle has prompted attempts to increase bladder capacity with β-adrenergic stimulation. Such stimulation can cause significant increases in the capacity of animal bladders, which contain a moderate density of β-adrenergic receptors.[37] In vitro studies show a strong dose-related relaxant effect of β_2 agonists on the bladder body of rabbits, but little effect on the bladder base or proximal urethra. Terbutaline, in oral dosages of 5 mg TID has been reported to have a "good clinical effect" in some patients with urgency and urgency incontinence, but no significant effect on the bladders of neurologically normal humans without voiding difficulty.[38] Although these results are compatible with those in other organ systems (β-adrenergic stimulation causes no acute change in total lung capacity in normal humans while it does favorably affect patients with bronchial asthmas), few adequate studies are available on the effects of β-adrenergic stimulation in patients with detrusor hyperactivity. Lindholm and Lose[39] used 5 mg TID of terbutaline in eight women with motor and seven with sensory urge incontinence. After 3 months of treatment, 14 patients claimed beneficial effects, and 12 became subjectively continent. In 6 of 8 cases, the detrusor became stable on cystometry. Nine patients had transient side effects, including palpitations, tachycardia, and/or hand tremor, and in three of these, side effects continued but were acceptable. In one patient the drug was discontinued because of severe adverse symptoms. Gruneberger[40] reported that, in a double-blind study, clenbuterol had a good therapeutic effect in 15 of 20 with motor urge incontinence. Unfavorable results of β agonist usage for bladder hyperactivity were published by Castleden and Morgan[41] and Naglo et al.[42]

α-Adrenergic Antagonists

α-Adrenergic blocking agents have also been used to treat both bladder and outlet abnormalities in patients with so-called "autonomous" bladders.[43] These include voiding dysfunctions resulting from myelodysplasia, sacral spinal cord or infrasacral neural injury, and radical pelvic surgery. Decreased bladder compliance is often a clinical problem in such patients, and this, along with a fixed urethral sphincter tone, results in the paradoxical occurrence of both storage and emptying failure. Norlen[43] has summarized the supporting evidence for the success of α-adrenolytic treatment in these patients. Andersson et al.[44] used prazosin (Minipress) in such patients and found maximum urethral pressure during filling was decreased while "autonomous waves" were reduced. McGuire and Savastano[45] reported that phenoxybenzamine decreased filling cystometric pressure in the decentralized primate bladder. More recently Amark and Nergardh[46] reported that, in children with myelodysplasia, alpha blockade not only decreased urethral tone, but bladder tone and hyperactivity as well. Swierzewski et al.[47] studied the use of a 5 mg daily dose of terazosin (Hytrin) in 12 spinal cord injured patients who were candidates for cystoplasty because of decreased bladder compliance. Detrusor compliance improved in all patients, and bladder pressure at capacity decreased by a mean of 36 cm H_2O. The maximum safe volume stored at a detrusor pressure of 40 cm of water, increased by a mean of 157 ml.

α-Adrenergic blockage can decrease bladder contractility in patients with non-neurogenic voiding dysfunction as well. Jensen[2–4] reported an increase in "α-adrenergic effect" in bladders characterized as "uninhibited." Short- and long-term prazosin administration increased capacity and decreased the amplitude of contractions.

Tricyclic Antidepressants

Many clinicians have found tricyclic antidepressants, particularly imipramine hydrochloride, to be especially useful agents for facilitating urine storage, both by decreasing bladder contractility and increasing outlet resistance.[48] These agents have been the subject of a voluminous amount of highly sophisticated pharmacological investigation to determine the mechanisms of action responsible for their varied effects.[49,50] Most data have been accumulated as a result of trying to explain the antidepressant properties of these agents and thus primarily from CNS tissue. All of these agents possess varying degrees of at least three major pharmacological actions: (1) they have central and peripheral anticholinergic effects at some, but not all, sites; (2) they block the active transport system in the presynaptic nerve ending which is responsible for the reuptake of the released amine neurotransmitters norepinephrine and serotonin; and (3) they are sedatives, an action which occurs presumably on a central basis, but is perhaps related to antihistiminic properties (at H_1 receptors, although they also antagonize H_2 receptors to some extent). There is also evidence that they desensitize at least some α_2 adrenoceptors and some β adrenoceptors. Paradoxically, they also have been shown to block some α and serotonin-1 receptors. *Imipramine* has prominent systemic anticholinergic effects, but has only a weak antimuscarinic effect on bladder smooth muscle.[51] A strong direct inhibitory effect on bladder smooth muscle does exist, however, which is neither anticholinergic nor adrenergic.[52,53] This may be due to a local anesthetic-like action at the nerve terminals in the adjacent effector membrane, an effect that seems to occur also in cardiac muscle or to an inhibition of the participation of Ca in the excitation–contraction coupling process.[54] Direct evidence to suggest that the effect of imipramine on norepinephrine reuptake occurs on lower urinary tract tissue as well as brain tissue has been provided by Foreman and McNulty[55] in the rabbit. An enhanced α-adrenergic effect in the smooth muscle of the bladder base and proximal urethra, where α receptors outnumber β receptors, is generally considered to be the mechanism whereby imipramine increases outlet resistance. Attempting to correlate clinical effects with mechanisms of action, one might also postulate a β receptor–induced decrease in bladder body contractility if peripheral blockade of norepinephrine reuptake does occur there as well, due to the increased concentration of β over α-adrenergic receptors in that area.

Clinically, imipramine (Tofranil, others) seems to be effective in decreasing bladder contractility and in increasing outlet resistance.[56–60] Castleden et al.[60] began therapy in elderly patients with detrusor instability with a single 25-mg nighttime dose of imipramine, which was increased every third day by 25 mg until either the patient was continent, had side effects, or a dose of 150 mg was reached. Six of ten patients became continent, and, in those who underwent repeated cystometry, bladder capacity increased by a mean of 105 ml and bladder pressure at capacity decreased by a mean of 18 cm H_2O. Maximum urethral pressure (MUP) increased by a mean of 30 cm H_2O. Our usual adult dose for voiding dysfunction is 25 mg QID; less frequent administration is possible because of the drug's long half-life. Half that dose is given in elderly patients, in whom the drug half-life may be prolonged. In our experience, the effects of imipramine on the lower urinary tract are often additive to those of the atrophine-like agents, and consequently a combination of imipramine and an antimuscarinic or an antispasmodic is sometimes especially useful for decreasing bladder contractility. If imipramine is used in conjunction with an atropine-like agent, it should be noted that the anticholinergic side effects of the drugs may be additive.

Doxepin (Sinequan) is another tricyclic antidepressant which was found to be more potent, using in vitro rabbit bladder strips, than other tricyclic compounds with respect to antimuscarinic and musculotropic relaxant activity.[53] Lose et al.[61] in a randomized double-blind crossover study of female with involuntary bladder contractions and either frequency, urgency, or urge incontinence, found that this agent caused a significant decrease over control in nighttime frequency and nighttime incontinence episodes, and a near significant decrease in urine loss (pad weighing test), and in the cystometric parameters of first sensation and maximum bladder capacity (MBC). The dosage of doxepin utilized was either a single 50-mg bedtime dose or this dose plus an additional 25 mg in the morning. The number of daytime incontinence episodes decreased in both doxepin and placebo groups, and the difference was not statistically significant. Doxepin treatment was preferred by 14 patients, while two preferred placebo. Three patients had no preference. Of the 14 patients who stated a preference for doxepin, 12 claimed that they became continent during treatment, while two claimed improvement; the two patients who preferred placebo claimed improvement. The AHCPR guidelines combine results for imipramine and doxepin, citing only three randomized controlled trials, with an unknown percent of female patients. Percent cures (all figures refer to percent drug effect *minus* percent effect on placebo) are listed as 31%, percent reduction in urge incontinence as 20–77%, and percent side effects as 0–70%.[6]

When used in the large doses employed for antidepressant effects, the most frequent side effects of the tricyclic antidepressants are those attributable to their systemic anticholinergic activity.[49,50] Allergic phenomena, including rash, hepatic dysfunction, obstructive jaundice, and a granulocytosis may also occur, but rarely. CNS side effects may include weakness, fatigue, parkinsonian effect, a fine tremor noted most in the upper extremities, a manic or schizophrenic picture, and sedation, probably from an antihistaminic effect. Postural hypotension may also be seen, presumably on the basis of selective blockade (a paradoxical effect of α_1-adrenergic receptors in some vascular smooth muscle. They can also produce arrhythmias, and interact in deleterious ways with other drugs, and so caution must be observed in their use in patients with cardiac disease.[49] Whether cardiotoxicity will prove to be a legitimate concern in patients receiving the smaller doses (than for treatment of depression) for lower urinary tract dysfunction remains to be seen, but is a potential matter of concern. Consultation with a patient's internist or cardiologist is always helpful before instituting such therapy in questionable situations. The use of imipramine is contraindicated in patients receiving monoamine oxidase inhibitors, as severe CNS toxicity can be precipitated, including hyperpyrexia, seizures, and coma. Some potential side effects of the antidepressants may be especially significant for the elderly, specifically weakness, fatigue, and postural hypotension. If imipramine or any of the tricyclic antidepressants is to be prescribed for the treatment of voiding dysfunction, the patient should be thoroughly informed of the fact that this is *not* the usual indication for this drug, and that potential side effects exist. Reports of significant side effects (severe abdominal distress, nausea, vomiting, headache, lethargy, and irritability) following abrupt cessation of high doses of imipramine in children would suggest that the drug should be discontinued gradually, especially in patients receiving high doses.

Dimethyl Sulfoxide (DMSO)

Sant[62] has summarized the pharmacology and clinical usage of intravesical DMSO, and has tabulated good to excellent results in 50–90% of a collected series of patients treated with intravesical instillation for interstitial cystitis. However, DMSO has not been shown to be useful in the treatment of detrusor hyperreflexia or instability or in any patients with urgency/frequency but without interstitial cystitis.

Increasing Bladder Capacity by Decreasing Sensory (Afferent) Input

Decreasing afferent input peripherally would be the ideal treatment for sensory urgency and for instability or hyperreflexia in a bladder with relatively normal elastic/viscoelastic properties in which the sensory afferents constituted the first limb in the abnormal micturition reflex. Maggi[63,64] has written extensively about the potential for treatment, specifically with reference to the properties of capsaicin, an irritant and algogenic compound obtained from hot red peppers which has highly selective effects on a subset of mammalian sensory neurons, including polymodal receptors and warm thermoreceptors.[65] Systemic and topical capsaicin produces a reversible antinociceptive and anti-inflammatory action after an initially undesirable algesic effect. Local or topical application blocks C-fiber conduction and inactivates neuropeptide release from peripheral nerve endings, accounting for local antinociception and reduction of neurogenic inflammation. With intravesical administration the potential advantage is a lack of systemic side effects. The actions are highly specific when applied locally—the compound affects primarily small-diameter nociceptive afferents, leaving the sensations of touch and pressure unchanged, although heat (not cold) perception may be reduced. Motor fibers are not affected.[66] The effects are reversible, although it is unknown whether initial levels of sensitivity are regained. Craft and Porreca[66] list intravesical doses for the rat at 0.03—10.0 μM for 15–30 minutes and, for the human, up to a 1–2 mM dose.

Maggi[64] reviewed the therapeutic potential of capsaicin-like molecules. Intravestical instillation of capsaicin into human bladder produced a concentration-dependent decrease in the volume at first desire to void, decreased bladder capacity, and a warm burning sensation. Concentrations used were doses of 0.01, 1.0 and 10 μM, administered in ascending order at 10 to 15 min intervals as constant infusions of 20 ml/min until micturition. Five capsaicin-treated patients with "hypersensitive disorders" reported either a complete disappearance (4) or marked attenuation (1) of their symptoms, beginning 2–3 days after administration and lasting 4–16 days. After that time symptoms gradually reappeared, but were not worse. Fowler et al.[65] reported on the use of capsaicin in 14 patients with detrusor hyperactivity, 12 with spinal cord disease. Low concentrations (0.1–10 μM/L) had no effect on bladder capacity or hyperactivity. The dose suggested was 100 ml of either 1 mmol/L (0.3 g/L) or 1 mmol/L dissolved in 30% alcohol in saline introduced intravesically with a balloon catheter (to prevent urethral leakage) and left in place for 30 min. All patients with bladder sensation reported immediate suprapubic burning that lasted 5–10 min. All reported initial deterioration of their symptoms for a period of 1–14 days followed by a clinical improvement or a return to their previous state. An improvement in some aspect of bladder behavior was seen in nine patients, great improvement (increase in bladder capacity from 127 to 404 ml with continence between CIC in five. Systemic side effects did not occur. The longest follow-up was 20 months in a patient who was retreated at 3, 12, and 20 months. It is unclear from the report what the exact effects on compliance were, but the results certainly deserve the authors' designation of "promising" for the treatment of intractable hyperreflexia and incontinence and seem to confirm that capsaicin-sensitive afferents exist in the human bladder and become functionally significant in the detrusor hyperreflexia seen secondary to spinal disease.

Increasing Outlet Resistance

α-Adrenergic Agonists

The bladder neck and proximal urethra contain a preponderance of α-adrenergic receptor sites, which, when stimulated, produce smooth muscle contraction.[1,67] The static infusion urethral pressure profile is altered by such stimulation, which produces an increase in maximum urethral pressure (MUP) and maximum urethral closure pressure (MUCP). Various orally administered pharmacologic agents are available which produce α-adrenergic stimulation. Generally, outlet resistance is increased to a variable degree by such an action. Potential side effects of all of these agents include blood pressure elevation, anxiety, and insomnia due to stimulation of the CNS, headache, tremor, weakness, palpitation, cardiac arrhythmias, and respiratory difficulties. They all should be used with caution in patients with hypertension, cardiovascular disease, or hyperthyroidism.[68]

Ephedrine is a noncatecholamine sympathomimetic agent which enhances release of norepinephrine from sympathetic neurons and directly stimulates both α- and β-adrenergic receptors.[68] The oral adult dosage is 25–50 mg QID. Some tachyphylaxis develops to its peripheral actions, probably as a result of depletion of norepinephrine stores. *Pseudoephedrine,* a steroisomer of ephedrine, is used for similar indications with similar precautions. The adult dosage is 30–60 mg QID, and the 30-mg dose form is available in the United States without prescription. Diokno and Taub[69] reported a "good to excellent" result in 27 of 38 patients with sphincteric incontinence treated with ephedrine sulfate. Beneficial effects were most often achieved in those with minimal to moderate wetting, and little benefit was achieved in patients with severe stress incontinence. A dose of 75–100 mg of norephedrine chloride has been shown to increase MUP and MUCP in women with urinary stress incontinence.[70] At a 300-ml bladder volume, MUP rose from 82 to 110 cm H_2O, and MUCP rose from 63 to 93 cm H_2O. The functional profile length did not change significantly. Obrink and Bunne,[71] however, noted that 100 mg of norephedrine chloride BID did not improve severe stress incontinence sufficiently to offer it as an alternative to surgical treatment. They further noted in their group of ten such patients that the MUCP was not influenced at rest or with stress at low or moderate bladder volumes. Lose and Lindholm[72] treated 20 women with stress incontinence with norfenefrine, an α agonist, given as a slow-release tablet. Nineteen patients reported reduced urinary leakage; 10 reported no further stress incontinence. MUCP increased in 16 patients during treatment, the mean rise being 53 to 64 cm H_2O. It is interesting and perplexing that most patients reported an effect only after 14 days of treatment. This delay is difficult to explain on the basis of drug action, unless one postulates a change in the number of α receptors or in their sensitivity.

Phenylpropanolamine hydrochloride (PPA) shares the pharmacologic properties of ephedrine and is approximately equal in peripheral potency while causing less central stimulation.[68] It is available in 25- and 50-mg tablets, 75-mg time-release capsules, and is a component of numerous proprietary mixtures marketed for the treatment of nasal and sinus congestion (usually in combination with an H_1 antihistamine drug) and as an appetite suppressant. Utilizing doses of 50 mg TID, Awad et al.[73] found that 11 of 13 females and 6 of 7 males with stress incontinence were significantly improved after 4 weeks of therapy. MUCP increased from a mean of 47 to 72 cm H_2O in patients with an empty bladder and from 43 to 58 in patients with a full bladder. Using a capsule which contained 50 mg of PPA, 8 mg of chlorpheniramine (an antihistamine), and 2 mg of isopropamide (an antimuscarinic), Stewart et al.[74] found that, of 77 women with stress urinary incontinence, 18 were completely cured with one sustained-release capsule BID. Twenty-eight patients were "much better," six were "slightly better," and 25 were no better. In 11 men with post-prostatectomy stress incontinence, the numbers in the corresponding categories were 1, 2, 1, and 7. The formulation of Ornade has now been changed, and each capsule of drug contains 75 mg of PPA and 12 mg of chlorpheniramine. Collste and Linokog[75] reported on a group of 24 women with stress urinary incontinence (SUI) treated with PPA or placebo with a crossover after 2 weeks. Severity was graded 1 (slight) or 2 (moderate). Average MUCP overall increased significantly with PPA compared to placebo (Pl) (48–55 versus 48–49 cm H_2O). This was significant in grade 2 but not grade 1 patients. The average number of leakage episodes per 48 hr was reduced significantly overall for PPA patients (5 to 2 versus 5 to 6). This was significant for grade 1 but not grade 2 patients. Subjectively 6 of 24 felt both PPA and Pl were ineffective. Of 18 of 24 reporting a subjective preference, 14 preferred PPA and 4 Pl. Improvements were rated subjectively as good, moderately good, and slight. Those obtained with PPA were significant versus placebo for the entire population and for both groups individually. The AHCPR guideline[6] reports eight randomized controlled trials with PPA 50 mg BID for SUI in females. Percent cures (all figures refer to percent effect on drug *minus* percent effect on placebo) and listed as 0–14, percent reduction in incontinence as 19–60, and percent side effects and percent dropouts as 5–33 and 0–4.3 respectively.

Some authors have emphasized potential complications of phenylpropanolamine. Baggioni et al.[76] emphasized the possibility of blood pressure elevation, especially in patients with autonomic impairment. Lasagna[77] has pointed out that prior reported blood pressure elevations were with a product that differed from American PPA and probably contained a different and much more potent isomer. He pointed out that even though a huge volume of PPA has been consumed for decongestant and anorectic purposes, the world literature has carried only a minimal number of possible toxic reactions, most of which have involved excessively high doses in combination medications. Liebson et al.[78] found no cardiovascular or subjective adverse effects with doses of 25 mg TID or a 75-mg sustained-release preparation in a population of 150 healthy normal volunteers. Blackburn et al.,[79] in a larger series of healthy subjects and using multiple over-the-counter formulations, concluded that there was a statistically significant but clinically unimportant pressor effect in the first 6 hr after administration of PPA and this was greater with a sustained-release preparation. Caution should still be exercised in individuals known to be significantly hypertensive and in the elderly, whose pharmacokinetics may be altered.

Although some clinicians have reported spectacular cure and improvement rates with α-adrenergic agonists and agents that produce an α-adrenergic effect in the outlet of patients with sphincteric urinary incontinence, our own experience coincides with those who report that such treatment with such agents often produces satisfactory or some improvement in mild cases, but rarely total dryness in cases of severe or even moderate stress incontinence. A clinical trial, where possible, is certainly worthwhile, however, especially in conjunction with pelvic floor physiotherapy/biofeedback.

β-Adrenergic Antagonists and Agonists

Theoretically, β-adrenergic blocking agents might be expected to "unmask" or potentiate an α-adrenergic effect, thereby increasing urethral resistance. Gleason et al.[80] reported success in training certain patients with stress urinary incontinence with propranolol, using oral doses of 10 mg QID. The beneficial effect became manifest only after 4–10 weeks of treatment. It is difficult to explain such a long delay in the onset of the therapeutic effect of incontinence. Kaisary[81] also reported success with propranolol in treating stress incontinence. Although such treatment has been suggested as alternative treatment to α agonists in patients with sphincteric incontinence and hypertension, few if any subsequent reports of such efficacy have appeared. Others have reported no significant changes in urethral profile pressures in normal women after β-adrenergic blockade.[82] Though 10 mg QID is a relatively small dose of propranolol, it should be recalled that the major potential side effects of the drug are related to its therapeutic β-blocking effects. Heart failure may develop, as well as an increase in airway resistance, and asthma is a contraindication to its use. Abrupt discontinuation may precipitate an exacerbation of anginal attacks and rebound hypertension.

β-Adrenergic stimulation is generally conceded to decrease urethral pressure (see ref. 1 for references), but β$_2$ agonists have been reported to *increase* the contractility of fast-contracting striated muscle fibers (extensor digitorum longus) from guinea pigs and suppress that of slow-contracting fibers (soleus).[83] Some β agonists also stimulate skeletal muscle hypertrophy, fast-twitch fibers more than slow-twitch.[84] Clenbuterol, a selective β$_2$ agonist, has been reported to potentiate, in a dose-dependent fashion, the field stimulation–induced contraction in isolated periurethral muscle preparation in the rabbit. The potentiation is greater than that produced by isoproterenol and is suppressed by propranolol.[85] These authors report an *increase* in urethral pressure with clinical use of clenbuterol and speculate on its promise for the treatment of sphincteric incontinence. Yamanishi et al.[86] reports an inotropic effect of clenbuterol and terbutaline on the fatigued striated urethral sphincter in female dogs, abolished by β blockade. They also cite their own experience and that of others which suggest effectiveness of clenbuterol in the treatment of stress incontinence.

Estrogens

Although estrogens were recommended for the treatment of urinary incontinence in females as early as 1941,[87] there is a great deal of controversy over their utility and benefit/risk ratio for this indication.

Much attention has been paid to the innervation, physiology, and pharmacology of the smooth muscle of the uterus. Estrogens have been found to effect many related properties including excitability, neuronal influences on the muscle, receptor density and sensitivity, and transmitter metabolism, especially in adrenergic nerves. The urethra (and trigone) are embryologically related to the uterus, and significant work has also been done on the effects estrogenic hormones on the lower urinary tract. Hodgson et al.[88] reported that the sensitivity of the rabbit urethra to α-adrenergic stimulation was estrogen-dependent; castration caused a decreased sensitivity, and treatment with low levels of estrogen reversed this. Larsson et al.[89] reported that estrogen treatment of the isolated female rabbit urethra caused an increased sensitivity to norepinephrine. The mechanism was postulated to be related to a more than twofold increase in the α-adrenergic stimulation, but that this did not occur in the rabbit or guinea pig. Bump and Friedman[90] reported that sex hormone replacement with estrogen, but not testosterone, enhanced the urethral sphincter mechanism in the castrate female baboon by effects which were unrelated to skeletal muscle. They added that these effects might not be related just to changes in the urethral smooth musculature, but to changes in the urethral mucosa, submucosal vascular plexus, and connective tissue.

Estrogen therapy certainly seems capable of facilitating urinary storage in some postmenopausal female patients. Whether this effect is related to just changes in the autonomic innervation or receptor content of function of the smooth muscle, or to changes in estrogen binding sites,[91] or to changes in the vascular and/or connective tissue elements of the urethral wall has not been settled. Batra et al.[92] have shown that low doses of estradiol and estratriol increased blood perfusion into the urethra (and also vagina and uterus) of oophorectomized mature female rabbits. After menopause, urethral pressure parameters normally decrease somewhat,[93] and though this is generally conceded to be related in some way to decreased estrogenic levels, whether the actual changes occur in smooth muscle, blood circulation, the supporting tissues, or the "mucosal seal mechanism" is still largely a matter of speculation. Versi et al.[94] describe a positive correlation between skin collagen content, which does decline with declining estrogen status, and parameters of the urethral pressure profile, suggesting that estrogen effect on the urethra may be predicted, at least in part, by changes in the collagen component. Eika et al.[95] reported that bladders from ovarectomized rats weighed less and had a higher collagen content and decreased atropine resistance than controls, and that estrogen substitution reversed these parameters.

Raz et al.[96] found that a daily dose of 2.5 mg of premarin (conjugated estrogens) improved stress incontinence and increased urethral pressures in 65% of postmenopausal patients, effects that they attributed to mucosal proliferation with a consequently improved "mucosal seal effect" and to enhancement of the α-adrenergic contractile response of urethral smooth musculature to endogenous catecholamines. Schreiter et al.[97] reported similar benefits after 10 days of treatment with daily divided doses of 6 mg of estriol. They also presented evidence that the effects of estrogen and of exogenous α-adrenergic stimulation were additive. In one of the first studies to present some quantitative data on estrogen, Rud[98] reported the effects of 4 mg daily doses of estradiol and 8 mg daily doses of estriol on 30 women, average age 61, 24 of whom had SUI. Small but statistically significant changes occurred in the MUP (59–63 cm H_2O), functional urethral length (25–28 mm), and actual urethral length (33–37 mm). No statistically significant change occurred in urethral closure pressure (37–39 cm H_2O). Eight of the 24 incontinent patients experienced subjective and objective improvement, nine experienced subjective improvement only, and seven experienced neither subjective nor objective improvement. There was no correlation between subjective or objective improvement and urodynamic parameters. However, of 18 patients in whom pressure transmission to the urethra was recorded during cough, seven improved. All of these had subjective improvement and five were shown to be objectively dry. Rud pointed out that it is hard to believe that the small changes in urodynamic measurements, even though statistically significant, were directly related to resumption of continence and noted that the increased pressure transmission ratio might be due to factors outside the urethra—either in the striated musculature of the pelvic floor or in the periurethral vasculature or supporting tissues. Rud[93] also studied profilometry during the menstrual cycle in six females. There was no change in any profilometric values during the menstrual cycle and no correlation between estrogen levels and MUP. It may be, as suggested, that at physiologic levels estrogens have little influence on urodynamic measurements related to continence, and that only pharmacologic doses cause urodynamically significant changes. Pharmacologic doses might also alter responses to other exogenous autonomic stimulation, particularly α-adrenergic, as laboratory experiments would suggest.

Beisland et al.[99] carried out a randomized open, comparative crossover trial in 20 postmenopausal women with urethral sphincteric insufficiency. Both oral PPA 50 mg BID and estriol vaginal suppositories, 1 mg daily, significantly increased the MUCP and the continence area on profilometry. PPA was clinically more effective than estriol, but not sufficient to obtain complete continence. However, with combined treatment, eight patients became completely continent, nine were considerably improved, and only one patient remained unchanged. Two patients dropped out of the study because of side effects. Bhata et al.[100] used 2 gm daily of conjugated estrogen vaginal cream for 6 weeks in 11 postmenopausal women with SUI. Six were cured or improved significantly. Favorable response was correlated with increased closure pressure and increased pressure transmission. In an accompanying article, Karram et al.[101] reported that estrogen administration to six women, with premature ovarian failure (but *without* lower urinary tract problems) did not produce any change in urethral pressure, functional length, or cystometric parameters. However, a significant increase in pressure transmission ratio to the proximal and midurethra was noted after vaginal estrogen (89 to 109 and 86 to 100% respectively), but not after oral estrogen, even though serum E2 levels and cytologic changes were similar with the two modes of administration. Negative effects on the effect of estrogen alone on stress incontinence were reported by Walter et al.,[102] Hilton and Stanton,[103] and Samsioe et al.,[104] but in each of these studies urge symptomatology was favorably affected. Cardozo,[105] in a review article, concluded that "there is no conclusive evidence that estrogen even improves, let alone cures, stress incontinence," although it "apparently alleviates urgency, urge incontinence, frequency, nocturia and dysuria."

Kimm and Lindskog[106] described the results of treatment of 36 postmenopausal women with SUI with oral estriol and PPA, alone and in combination, in a double-blind trial, but after a 4-week run-in period with PPA. Although some of the data are difficult to interpret, the authors concluded that PPA alone and PPA plus estriol raised the intraurethral pressure and reduced urinary loss by 35% (significant) in a standardized physical strain test. Leakage episodes and amounts were significantly reduced by estriol and PPA given separately (28%) or as combined therapy (40%). The authors found no evidence for a synergistic effect, but did indicate an additive effect was present. Walter et al.[102] completed a complicated but logical study on 28 (out of 38 original subjects) postmenopausal women with SUI. After 4 weeks of placebo (Pl) run-in, patients were randomized to oral estriol (E3) or PPA alone for 4 weeks, then to combined therapy for 4 weeks. In the group which sequentially received P-PPA-PPA/E3, the percentages reporting cure/improvement respectively were 0/13, 13/20, 21/14. In the group, receiving P-E3-E3/PPA the corresponding percentages were 0/0, 14/29, 64/7. Objective parameters showed the following. The number of leak episodes per 24 hr in patients treated with PPA first showed a 31% decrease ($\sim$3–2) compared to placebo (Pl < 0.003). For those treated with E3 first the change was not significant ($\sim$ 1.5–0.8). Combined treatment produced a mean decrease of 48% over placebo. There was a greater effect with E/PLPA than PPA/E. Pad weights (gm in 1-hr test) decreased significantly with PPA alone ($\sim$ 27 to 6) but there was no difference between PPA and PPA/E3. E3 alone significantly decreased pad weights ($\sim$ 47 to 15). Although E3/PLPA was not significantly different, there was a further numerical loss from $\sim$ 15 to 3. The overall conclusions were that E3 and PPA are each effective in treating SUI in postmenopausal females, and, based on subjective data, combined therapy is better than either alone. This was substantiated by a significant decrease in the number of leak episodes in the patients in whom E3 was given before PPA, but not confirmed statistically by pad weighing tests.

Hilton et al.[107] published the results of a double-blind study of 60 (originally) postmenopausal women with SUI treated for 4 weeks with oral and vaginal estrogen alone and in combination with PPA. There were six groups in this study: vaginal estrogen (VE)/PPA; VE/oral placebo (OP); oral estrogen (OE)/PPA; OE/OP; vaginal placebo (VP)/PPA; and VP/OP. Subjective symptoms and reported pads per day (PPD) decreased in *all* groups; the greatest reduction was in those treated with VE, although the reduction in groups 1, 2, 4, and 6 were *all* significant. Objective pad weight after exercise test showed a slight decrease in all groups except the double placebo one. Reduction was maximal in the VE/PPA group (22 to 8 gm), but the pretreatment values for PPD and pad weight varied greatly (< 0.5 PPD to $\sim$ 3.5; < 5 gm to 22). There was no change in cystometry or urethral profilometry, either resting or stress.

Sessions et al.[108] review the benefits and risks of estrogen replacement therapy. Improvement in vasomotor symptomatology and osteoporosis prevention are well established. There is also substantial evidence for a decreased risk of cardiovascular disease, perhaps due to an effect on the lipid profile. There is little question, however, that unopposed estrogen use in those with an intact uterus increases the risk of endometrial cancer. Progestin treatment exerts a protective effect, and the daily administration of an estrogen and progestin provides an attractive alternative because of a lack of withdrawal bleeding (with sequential therapy) and consequent increased patient compliance. Whether progestin administration will adversely affect the results of estrogen treatment of SUI is unknown but must be considered (see prior discussion of the effect of progestin on urethral responses and flowmetry). Progestins may also cause mastalgia, edema, and bloating. It is concluded, further, that there is no evidence for an increase in thromboembolism or hypertension with estrogen replacement. Transdermal administration of estrogen avoids any theoretical problems associated with the first-pass effect through the liver with oral administration (alteration in clotting factors and increase in renin substrate). Evidence does suggest an association between breast cancer and estrogen replacement therapy, but only for those receiving such therapy for more than 15 years. A preventive role of progestin in this regard is controversial, as is the dose of estrogen necessary to produce this effect. As to the type of estrogen preparation preferred, transdermal seems as effective as oral and subcutaneous implants seem to produce physiologic serum levels. Percutaneous and intramuscular seem to produce variable serum levels. Vaginal creams are said to produce variable serum levels but physiologic E_2:E_1 ratios.[108] We agree that "hands on" application to the "affected area" may have a psychological benefit, however, as well, as suggested by Murray.[109]

Circumventing the Problem

ANTIDIURETIC HORMONE-LIKE AGENTS   The synthetic antidiuretic hormone peptide analogue (DDAVP; 1-(3-mercaptopriopionic)-8-D-arginine vasopressin monoacetate trihydrate) has been utilized for the symptomatic relief of refractory nocturnal enuresis in both children and adults.[110,111] The drug can conveniently be administered by intranasal spray at bedtime (dose 10–40 μg) and effectively suppress urine production for 7–10 hr. Its clinical long-term safety has been established by continued use in patients with diabetes insipidus. At present, this novel circumventive approach to the treatment of urinary frequency and incontinence has been largely restricted to those with nocturnal enuresis and diabetes insipidus. Recently, suggestions have been made that DDAVP might be useful in patients with refractory nocturnal frequency and incontinence, but who do not fall into the category of primary nocturnal enuresis or decreased antidiuretic hormone secretion. Kinn and Larsson[112] report that micturition frequency "decreased significantly" in 13 patients with multiple sclerosis and urge incontinence treated with oral tablets of desmopressin and that less leakage occurred. The actual approximate verge change in the number of voiding during the 6 hr after drug intake was 3.2–2.5. Eckford et al.[113] showed a numerically small but statistically significant decrease in nocturnal urinary frequency, nocturnal urine volume, and percent of urine passed at night in a group of patients with multiple sclerosis treated with DDAVP. Following the study "the majority" continued to use the drug, but many for just "spot" usage—to avoid social inconvenience or during an exacerbation of their voiding symptoms.

REFERENCES

1. Andersson KE: Pharmacology of lower urinary tract smooth muscles and penile erectile tissues. *Pharmacol Rev* 45:253, 1993.

2. Jensen D Jr: Pharmacological studies of the uninhibited neurogenic bladder. *Acta Neurol Scand* 64:175, 1981.

3. Jensen D Jr: Altered adrenergic innervation in the uninhibited neurogenic bladder. *Scand J Urol Nephrol* 60:61, 1981.

4. Jensen D Jr: Uninhibited neurogenic bladder treated with prazosin. *Scand J Urol Nephrol* 15:229, 1981.

5. Brown JH: Atropine, scopolamine and related antimuscarinic drugs. In Gilman AG, Rall TW, Nies AS, et al (eds): *Goodman and Gilman's The Pharmacological Basis of Therapeutics,* ed 8. New York, Pergamon Press, 1990, pp 150–165.

6. Urinary Incontinence Guideline Panel. *Urinary Incontinence in Adults: Clinical Practice Guideline.* AHCPR Pub. No. 92-0038. Rockville, MD: Agency for Health Care Policy and Research, Public Health Service, U.S. Department of Health and Human Services, March, 1992.

7. Lau W, Szilagyi M: A pharmacological profile of glycopyrrolate: interactions at the muscarinic acetylcholine receptor. *Gen Pharmacol* 23:1165, 1992.

8. Tonini M, Rizzi CA, Perrucca E, et al: Depressant action of oxybutynin on the contractility of intestinal and urinary tract smooth muscle. *J Pharm Pharmacol* 39:103, 1987.

9. Kachur JF, Peterson JS, Carter JP, et al: R and S enantiomers or oxybutynin: pharmacological effects in guinea pig bladder and intestine. *J Pharmacol Exp Ther* 247:867, 1988.

10. Thompson I, Lauvetz R: Oxybutynin in bladder spasm, neurogenic bladder and enuresis. *Urology* 8:452, 1976.

11. Andersson KE: Current concepts in the treatment of disorders of micturition. *Drugs* 35:477, 1988.

12. Moisey C, Stephenson T, Brendler C: The urodynamic and subjective results of treatment of detrusor instability with oxybutynin chloride: *Br J Urol* 52:472, 1980.

13. Hehir M, Fitzpatrick JM: Oxybutynin and the prevention of urinary incontinence in spina bifida. *Eur Urol* 11:254, 1985.

14. Gajewski JB, Awad JA: Oxybutynin versus propantheline in patients with multiple sclerosis and detrusor hyperreflexia. *J Urol* 135:966, 1986.

15. Holmes DM, Monty FJ, Stanton SL: Oxybutynin versus propantheline in the management of detrusor instability. A patient regulated variable dose trial. *Br J Obstet Gynecol* 96:607, 1989.

16. Thuroff J, Bunke B, Ebner A, et al: Randomized double-blind multicenter trial on treatment of frequency, urgency and incontinence related to detrusor hyperactivity: oxybutynin vs propantheline vs placebo. *J Urol* 145:813, 1991.

17. Zorzitto ML, Jewett MA, Fernie, et al: Effectiveness of propantheline bromide in the treatment of geriatric patients with detrusor instability. *Neurourol Urodyn* 5:133, 1986.

18. Ouslander JG, Blaustein J, Connor H: P.II A habit training and oxybutynin for incontinence in nursing home patients: a placebo controlled trial. *J Am Geriatr Soc* 36:40, 1988.

19. Ouslander JG, Blaustein J, Connor A, et al: Pharmacokinetics and clinical effects of oxybutynin in geriatric patients. *J Urol* 140:47, 1988.

20. Kato K, Kitada S, Chun A, et al: In vitro intravesical instillation of anticholinergic antispasmodic and calcium blocking agents (rabbit whole bladder model). *J Urol* 141:1471, 1989.

21. Madersbacher H, Jilg G: Control of detrusor hyperreflexia by the intravesical instillation of oxybutynin hydrochloride. *Paraplegia* 19:84, 1991.

22. Weese DL, Roskamp DA, Leach GE, et al: Intravesical oxybutynin chloride: experience with 42 patients. *Urology* 41:527, 1993.

23. Fischer C, Diokno A, Lapides J: The anticholinergic effects of dicyclomine hydrochloride in uninhibited neurogenic bladder dysfunction. *J Urol* 120:328, 1978.

24. Beck RP, Amausch T, King C: Results in testing 210 patients with detrusor overactivity incontinence of urine. *Am J Obstet Gynecol* 125:593, 1976.

25. Awad S, Bryniak S, Downie JW, et al: The treatment of the uninhibited bladder with dicyclomine. *J Urol* 117:161, 1977.

26. Jonas U, Petri E, Kissal J: The effect of flavoxate on hyperactive detrusor muscle. *Eur Urol* 5:106, 1979.

27. Briggs RS, Castleden CM, Asher MJ: The effect of flavoxate on uninhibited detrusor contractions and urinary incontinence in the elderly. *J Urol* 123:656, 1980.

28. Chapple CR, Parkhouse H, Gardener C, et al: Double blind, placebo controlled, crossover study of flavoxate in the treatment of idiopathic detrusor instability. *Bri J Urol* 66:491, 1990.

29. Abrams P: Terodilene in clinical practice. *Urology* 36(suppl):60, 1990.

30. Peters D and Multicentre Study Group: Terodilene in the treatment of urinary frequency and motor urge incontinence, a controlled multicentre trial. *Scand J Urol Nephrol Suppl* 87:21, 1984.

31. Tapp A, Fall M, Norgaard J, et al: Terodilene: a dose titrated, multicenter study of the treatment of idiopathic detrusor instability in women. *J Urol* 142:1027, 1989.

32. Connolly MJ, Astridge PS, White EG, et al: torsade de pointes ventricular tachycardia and terodilene. *Lancet* 338:344 (Aug. 10), 1991.

33. Andersson KE: Clinical pharmacology of potassium channel openers. *Pharmacol Toxicol* 70:244, 1992.

34. Malmgren A, Andersson KE, Fovaeus M, et al: Effects of cromkalim and pinacidil on normal and hypertrophied rat detrusor in vitro. *J Urol* 143:828, 1990.

35. Hedlund H, Mattiasson A, Andersson KE: Lack of effect of pinacidil on detrusor instability in men with bladder outlet obstruction. *J Urol* 143:369A, 1990.

36. Nurse D, Restorick J, Mundy A: The effect of cromkalim on the normal and hyperreflexic human detrusor muscle. *Br J Urol* 68:27, 1991.

37. Wein AJ, Barrett DM: *Voiding Function and Dysfunction: A Logical and Practical Approach.* Chicago, Year Book Medical Publishers, 1988.

38. Norlen L, Sundin T, Waagstein F: Beta-adrenoceptor stimulation of the human urinary bladder in vivo. *Acta Pharmacol Toxicol* 43:5, 1978.

39. Lindholm P, Lose G: Terbutaline (Bricanyl) in the treatment of female urge incontinence. *Urol Int* 41:158, 1986.

40. Gruneberger A: Treatment of motor urge incontinence with clenbuterol and flavoxate hydrochloride. *Br J Obstet Gynecol* 91:275, 1984.

41. Castelden CM, Morgan B: The effect of beta adrenoceptor agonists on urinary incontinence in the elderly. *Br J Clin Pharmacol* 10:619, 1980.

42. Naglo AS, Nergardh A, Boreus LO: Influence of atropine and isoprenoline on detrusor hyperactivity in children with neurogenic bladder. *Scand J Urol Nephrol* 15:97, 1981.

43. Norlen L: Influence of the sympathetic nervous system on the lower urinary tract and its clinical implications. *Neurourol Urodyn* 1:129, 1982.

44. Andersson K, Ek A, Hedlund H, et al: Effects of prazosin on isolated human urethra and in patients with lower neuron lesions. *Invest Urol* 19:39, 1981.

45. McGuire E, Savastano J: Effect of alpha adrenergic blockade and anticholinergic agents on the decentralized primate bladder. *Neurourol Urodyn* 4:139, 1985.

46. Amark P, Nergardh A: Influence of adrenergic agonists and antagonists in urethral pressure, bladder pressure and detrusor hyperactivity in children with myelodysplasia. *Acta Pediatr Scand* 80:824, 1991.

47. Swierzewski S, Gormley EA, Belville WD, et al: The effect of terazosin on bladder function in the spinal cord injured patients. *J Urol* 151:951, 1994.

48. Barrett D, Wein AJ: Voiding dysfunction: diagnosis, classification and management. In Gillen-

water JY, Grayhack JT, Howards ST, et al (eds): *Adult and Pediatric Urology,* ed 2. St. Louis, Mosby-Year Book Medical Publishers, 1991, pp 1001–1099.

49. Baldessarini RJ: Drugs and the treatment of psychiatric disorders. In Gilman AG, Rall TW, Nies AS, et al (eds): *Goodman and Gilman's The Pharmacological Basis of Therapeutics,* ed 8. New York, Pergamon Press, 1990, pp 383–435.

50. Richelson E: Pharmacology of antidepressants—characteristics of the ideal drug. *Mayo Clin Proc* 69:1069, 1994.

51. Levin RM, Staskin DR, Wein AJ: Analysis of the anticholinergic and musculotropic effects of desmethylimipramine on the rabbit urinary bladder. *Urol Res* 11:259, 1983.

52. Olubadewo J: The effect of imipramine on rat detrusor muscle contractility. *Arch Int Pharmacodyn Ther* 145:84, 1980.

53. Levin RM, Wein AJ: Comparative effects of five tricyclic compounds on the rabbit urinary bladder. *Neurourol Urodyn* 3:127, 1984.

54. Malkowicz SB, Wein AJ, Ruggieri MR, et al: Comparison of calcium antagonist properties of antispasmodic agents. *J Urol* 138:667, 1987.

55. Foreman MM, McNulty AM: Alterations in K(+) evoked release of 3-H-Norepinephrine and contractile responses in urethral and bladder tissues induced by norepinephrine reuptake inhibition. *Life Sci* 53:193, 1993.

56. Cole A, Fried F: Favorable experiences with imipramine in the treatment of neurogenic bladder. *J Urol* 107:44, 1972.

57. Mahony D, Laferte F, Mahoney J: Observations on sphincter augmenting effect of imipramine in children with urinary incontinence. *Urology* 2:317, 1973.

58. Raezer DM, Benson GS, Wein AJ, et al: The functional approach to the management of the pediatric neuropathic bladder: a clinical study. *J Urol* 117:649, 1977.

59. Tulloch AGS, Creed KE: A comparison between propantheline and imipramine on bladder and salivary gland function. *Br J Urol* 51:359, 1979.

60. Castleden CM, George CF, Renwick AG, et al: Imipramine—a possible alternative to current therapy for urinary incontinence in the elderly. *J Urol* 125:218, 1981.

61. Lose G, Jorgenson L, Thunedborg P: Doxepin in the treatment of female detrusor overactivity: a randomized double-blind crossover study. *J Urol* 142:1024, 1989.

62. Sant G: Intravesical 50% dimethyl sulfoxide in the treatment of interstitial cystitis. *Urology* 4(suppl):17, 1987.

63. Maggi CA: Capsaicin and primary afferent neurons: from basic science to human therapy? *J Auton Nerv Syst.* 33:1, 1991.

64. Maggi CA: Therapeutic potential of capsaicin like molecules. *Life Sci* 51:1777, 1992.

65. Dray A: Mechanism of action of capsaicin like molecules on sensory neurons. *Life Sci* 51:1759, 1992.

66. Craft RM, Porreca F: Treatment parameters of desensitization to Capsaicin. *Life Sci* 51:1767, 1992.

67. Wein AJ, Levin RM, Barrett DM: Voiding function: relevant anatomy, physiology, and pharmacology. In Gillenwater JY, Grayhack JT, Howards ST, et al (eds): *Adult and Pediatric urology,* ed 2. St. Louis, Mosby-Year Book Medical Publishers, 1991, pp 933–999.

68. Hoffman BB, Lefkowitz RJ: Catecholamines and sympathomimetic drugs. In Gilman AG, Rall TW, Nies AS, et al (eds): *Goodman and Gilman's The Pharmacological Basis of Therapeutics,* ed 8. New York, Pergamon Press, 1990, pp 187–220.

69. Diokno A, Taub M: Ephedrine in treatment of urinary incontinence. *Urology* 5:624, 1975.

70. Ek A, Andersson KE, Gullberg B, et al: The effects of long-term treatment with norephedrine

on stress incontinence and urethral closure pressure profile. *Scand J Urol Nephrol* 12:105, 1978.

71. Obrink A, Bunne G: The effect of alpha adrenergic stimulation in stress incontinence. *Scand J Urol Nephrol* 12:205, 1978.

72. Lose G, Lindholm D: Clinical and urodynamic effects of norfenefrine in women with stress incontinence. *Urol Int* 39:298, 1984.

73. Awad S, Downie J, Kiruluta H: Alpha adrenergic agents in urinary disorders of the proximal urethra: I. Stress incontinence. *Br J Urol* 50:332, 1978.

74. Stewart B, Banowsky L, Montague D: Stress incontinence: conservative therapy with sympathomimetic drugs. *J Urol* 115:558, 1976.

75. Collste L, Linokog M: Phenylpropanolamine in treatment of female stress urinary incontinence: double-blind placebo controlled study in 24 patients. *Urology* 30:398, 1987.

76. Baggioni I, Onrot J, Stewart CK, et al: The potent pressor effect of phenylpropanolamine in patients with autonomic impairment. *JAMA* 258:236, 1987.

77. Lasagna L: Phenylpropanolamine and blood pressure. *JAMA* 253:2491, 1985.

78. Liebson I, Bigelow G, Griffiths RR, et al: Phenylpropanolamine: effects on subjective and cardiovascular variables at recommended over-the-counter dose levels. *J Clin Pharmacol* 27:685, 1987.

79. Blackburn GL, Morgan JP, Lavin PT, et al: Determinants of the pressor effect of phenylpropanolamine in healthy subjects. *JAMA* 261:3267, 1989.

80. Gleason D, Reilly R, Bottaccini M, et al: The urethral continence zone and its relation to stress incontinence. *J Urol* 112:81, 1974.

81. Kaisary AU: Beta adrenoceptor blockade in the treatment of female stress urinary incontinence. *J Urol* (Paris) 90:351, 1984.

82. Donker P, Van der Sluis C: Action of beta adrenergic blocking agents on the urethral pressure profile. *Urol Int* 31:6, 1976.

83. Fellenius E, Hedberg R, Holmberg E, et al: Functional and metabolic effects of terbutaline and propranolol in fast and slow contracting skeletal muscle in vitro. *Acta Physiol Scand* 109:89, 1980.

84. Kim YS, Sainz RD: Beta-adrenergic agonists and hypertrophy of skeletal muscles. *Life Sci* 50:397, 1992.

85. Kishimoto T, Morita T, Okamiya Y, et al: Effect of clenbuterol on contractile response in periurethral striated muscle of rabbits. *Tohoku J Exp Med* 165:243, 1991.

86. Yamanishi T, Yasuda K, Togo M, et al: Effects of beta-2 stimulants on contractility and fatigue of canine urethral sphincter. *J Urol* 151:1055, 1994.

87. Salmon UK, Walter RI, Geist SH: The use of estrogen in the treatment of dysuria and incontinence in post-menopausal women. *Am J Obstet Gynecol* 42:845, 1941.

88. Hodgson BT, Dumas S, Bolling DR, et al: Effect of estrogen on sensitivity of rabbit bladder and urethra to phenylephrine. *Invest Urol* 16:67, 1978.

89. Larsson B, Andersson KE, Batra S, et al: Effects of estradiol on norepinephrine-induced contraction, alpha adrenoreceptor number and norepinephrine content in the female rabbit urethra. *J Pharmacol Exp Ther* 229:557, 1984.

90. Bump RC, Friedman CI: Intraluminal urethral pressure measurements in the female baboon: effects of hormonal manipulation. *J Urol* 136:508, 1986.

91. Batra SC, Losif CS: Female urethra: a target for estrogen action. *J Urol* 129:418, 1983.

92. Batra S, Byellin L, Sjogren C: Increases in blood flow of the female rabbit urethra following low dose estrogens. *J Urol* 136:1360, 1986.

93. Rud T: Urethral pressure profile in continent women from childhood to old age. *Acta Obstet Gynecol Scand* 59:331, 1980.

94. Versi E, Cardozo L, Buncat L, et al: Correlation of urethral physiology and skin collagen in post menopausal women. *Br J Obstet Gynecol* 95:147, 1988.

95. Eika B, Salling LN, Christenson LL, et al: Long term observation of the detrusor smooth muscle in rats—its relationship to overiectomy and estrogen treatment. *Urol Res* 18:439, 1990.

96. Raz S, Ziegler M, Caine M: The role of female hormones in stress incontinence. *Proceedings of the 16th Congress of Société Internationale d'Urologie,* vol 1. Paris, 1973, pp 397–402.

97. Schreiter F, Fuchs P, Stockamp K: Estrogenic sensitivity of alpha receptors in the urethral musculature. *Urol Int* 31:13, 1976.

98. Rud T: The effects of estrogens and gestagens on the urethral pressure profile of urinary continent and stress incontinent women. *Acta Obstet Gynecol Scand* 59:265, 1980.

99. Beisland HO, Fossberg E, Moer A, et al: Urethral sphincteric insufficiency in postmenopausal females: treatment with phenylpropanolamine and estriol separately and in combination. *Urol Int* 39:211, 1984.

100. Bhatia NN, Bergman A, Karram MM: Effects of estrogen on urethral function in women with urinary incontinence. *Am J Obstet Gynecol* 160:176, 1989.

101. Karram MM, Yeko TR, Sauer MV, et al: Urodynamic changes following hormonal replacement therapy in women with premature ovarian failure. *Obstet Gynecol* 74:208, 1989.

102. Walter S, Wolf H, Barleto H, et al: Urinary incontinence in post menopausal women treated with estrogens. *Urol Int,* 33:135, 1978.

103. Hilton P, Stanton SL: The use of intravaginal estrogen cream in genuine stress incontinence. *Br J Obstet Gynecol* 90:940, 1983.

104. Samsioe G, Jansson I, Mellstrom D, et al: Occurrence, nature and treatment of urinary incontinence in a 70 year old female population. *Maturitas* 7:335, 1985.

105. Cardozo L: Role of estrogens in the treatment of female urinary incontinence. *J Am Geriatr Soc* 38:326, 1990.

106. Kinn AC, Lindskog M: Estrogen and phenylpropanolamine in combination for stress urinary incontinence in post-menopausal women. *Urology* 32:273, 1988.

107. Hilton P, Tweddel AL, Mayne C: Oral and intravaginal estrogens alone and in combination with alpha adrenergic stimulation in genuine stress incontinence. *Internat Urogynecol J* 1:90, 1990.

108. Sessions DR, Kelly AC, Jewelewicz R: Current concepts in estrogen replacement therapy in the menopause. *Fertil Steril* 59:277, 1993.

109. Murray K: Medical and surgical management of female voiding difficulty. In Drife JO, Hilton P, Stanton SL (eds): *Micturition.* London, Springer-Verlag, 1990, p 179.

110. Norgaard JP, Rillig S, Djurhuus JC: Nocturnal enuresis: an approach to treatment based on pathogenesis. *J Pediatr* 114:705, 1989.

111. Rew DA, Rundle JSH: Assessment of the safety of regular DDAVP therapy on primary nocturnal enuresis. *Br J Urol* 63:352, 1989.

112. Kinn AC, Larsson PO: Desmopressin: a new principle for symptomatic treatment of urgency and incontinence in patients with multiple sclerosis. *Scand J Urol Nephrol* 24:109, 1990.

113. Eckford SD, Swami KS, Jackson SR, et al: Desmopressin in the treatment of nocturia and enuresis in patients with multiple sclerosis. *Br J Urol* 74:733, 1994.

4

Pelvic Floor Exercise, Biofeedback, Electrical Stimulation, and Behavior Modification

Lauri J. Romanzi

In addition to surgical and pharmacologic methods for the treatment of incontinence, alternative methods are available for the appropriate, informed, and motivated patient and/or caretaker. While every incontinent patient may not prefer to invest the time and effort in nonsurgical methods, many suffering stress, urge, and mixed incontinence respond enthusiastically to the possibility of "self-help." Those suffering from sensory urgency and neurogenic bladder dysfunction may also benefit from pelvic floor exercises, biofeedback, electrical stimulation, and/or behavior modification. In 1992, the Agency for Health Care Policy and Research (under the auspices of the U.S. Department of Health and Human Services; AHCPR Pub. No. 92-0038 Rockville, MD) convened a panel of physicians, nurses, therapists, and consultants to evaluate the quality, appropriateness, and effectiveness of health care services as pertains to the diagnosis and treatment of urinary incontinence. Their effort concluded with the publication of *Urinary Incontinence in Adults: A Clinical Practice Guideline,* which concludes that "surgery, except in very specific cases, should be considered only after behavioral and pharmacologic interventions have been tried and that vigorous efforts should be made to educate the professional and lay public." Although one may reasonably argue that a mandated nonsurgical therapeutic trial may not represent optimal care for the individual patient, a working knowledge of these methods is prerequisite to providing full-scope care to those with bladder dysfunction.

PELVIC FLOOR EXERCISE

Pelvic floor exercise (PFE) entails the voluntary contraction of the pelvic floor musculature, or levator ani, in order to reduce or cure urinary dysfunction or incontinence. Exercise is typically done by the patient on a daily basis with office evaluation at regular intervals. PFE regimens generally involve rapid and sustained contractions in order to strengthen both the fast- and slow-twitch fibers found in the levator musculature. Instructing patients in the performance of pelvic floor exercises is a "hands on" effort, requiring individual instruction in order to assure proper muscle group isolation. One does the patient a disservice by simply giving her an instruction sheet without demonstrating the location and function of this muscle group at time of pelvic examination. In a demonstration of quick instruction during urodynamic testing, Bump et al. found that 25% of the women actually made a distinct Valsalva effort, which, if practiced regularly, may actually worsen pelvic floor tone and incontinence.[1] Bo et al. showed a significant difference in stress incontinent women undergoing 6 months of PFE either with or without intensive interval coaching with a physiotherapist, documenting the coached patients to be much more likely to report subjective cure (60%) than their uncoached counterparts (17%).[2] These results were supported by objective data on pad test and resting urethral closure pressure.

Patient Assessment

Prior to initiating PFE therapy, a baseline assessment of the pelvic floor is required. The patient is instructed in the anatomy and function of the pelvic floor; pelvic floor models or diagrams may prove useful. This is followed by physical evaluation in lithotomy position

Fig. 4.1. Pelvic Muscle Rating Scale (__/9)

	0	1	2	3
Pressure:	none	weak	moderate	strong
Duration:	none	<1 sec	1–5 sec	>5 sec
Displacement:	none	slt. ant.	whole ant.	gripped

Rating Scale Parameters:

a) Pressure: A flicker-like contraction that generates minimal or no resistance to digital retraction is termed *weak;* a contraction that generates definite but unsustained resistance to digital apposition is labeled *moderate;* a contraction that generates sustained resistance to digital apposition is labeled *strong.*

b) Duration: The baseline tone of the resting pelvic floor is assessed prior to the contraction. As the patient tightens the pelvic floor in a maximal effort, the amount of time the contraction takes (from intiation of contraction until return to baseline tone) is recorded as none, < 1 sec, 1–5 seconds or > 5 secs.

c) Displacement: Slight anterior displacement of the anterior wall will elevate and/or displace the distal portion of the examiner's fingers only; whole anterior displacement elevates and displaces the full length of the examiner's fingers without causing the fingers to override each other; gripped displacement will fully elevate and displace the examiner's fingers and cause the fingers to override.

and head elevated 30°. With two examining fingers in the vagina, the levator muscles are assessed bilaterally by palpation, being located at 5 and 7 o'clock just superior to the hymeneal ring. The patient is then instructed to contract these muscles. To assist proper muscle group isolation, various verbal cues can be tried, such as "squeeze as if you were trying to stop your urine stream" or "as if you were trying to prevent flatus" or "pull the examining fingers up into the vagina." A correctly performed pelvic floor contraction will be demonstrated by cephalad retraction of the perineum and anus, posterior rotation of the clitoris, and cephalad/anterior displacement of the examining fingers. Many patients unfamiliar with this maneuver will initially contract their abdominal wall and/or contract the buttocks or lower extremity adductors rather than the levator musculature. The examiner can observe this if the buttocks elevate, or if the other examining hand, resting lightly on the lower abdominal wall, palpates an abdominal wall contraction, or if the lower extremities actively adduct during the effort. The verbal cues and digital muscle identification can be repeated while reassuring the patient that many women are unable to identify the muscle group at first try. Once the examiner and patient are confident that the proper muscle group is being utilized, the patient is asked to contract as strongly as possible for as long as possible in order to assess the baseline pelvic floor function. This maximal effort is then rated according to a pelvic muscle rating scale.

A variety of pelvic muscle rating scales have been published.[3,4] We use a modification of a scale (Fig. 4.1) first published in 1986 by Worth et al. with a subsequent modification published in 1989 by Brink et al.[5,6] This scale incorporates objective (length of contraction in seconds) and semiobjective (anterior vaginal wall displacement and strength of contraction) data obtained during digital pelvic evaluation, with two examining fingers placed vaginally as during a standard gynecologic exam.

Once awareness and function of the muscle group have been established, the patient is instructed to perform a series of "quick flick," maximal and sustained contractions as part of a daily exercise regimen, initially done with examiner palpation and verbal feedback (Fig. 4.2). At our institution, patients are encouraged to return for weekly follow-up for a minimum of 1 month in order to assess progress and answer questions. Thereafter follow-up is done as frequently as possible; preferably monthly and no longer than every 3 months. If incontinence is the indication for therapy, voiding diaries are repeated at the follow-up intervals. We have found that the initial weekly follow-up is very difficult for both working women and housewives with small children; patient motivation and physician flexibility are prerequisite to a successful program.

History

First detailed by Arnold Kegel (hence the common name "Kegel exercises") in 1948, active rehabilitation of the levator musculature has found utility both as primary and adjunctive therapy.[7] In his initial description, Kegel described the use of a perineometer which measured vaginal pressure generated during pelvic floor contraction. This provided a method of biofeedback which he felt was particularly helpful for women with minimal voluntary control of the pelvic floor. His regimen involved pelvic floor contractions for 20-min periods three times daily, with the patient recording the maximum pressure generated each day. Using this method, he reported cure in 64 incontinent women, stating "There have been no failures when the condition was due primarily to relaxation or atrophy of the anterior vaginal muscles and the patient had at least partial control at times." Three years later he published a report of over 500 incontinent women, reporting an 84%

Fig. 4.2. Pelvic floor exercises

These exercises may be beneficial to women with stress and/or urge incontinence. They may also enhance sexual satisfaction. The exercises are designed to strengthen your internal vaginal muscles, also known as pelvic floor or levator muscles. You have already identified and contracted these muscles during your pelvic examination. They are the same muscles you use to "hold it" when you are on line for the bathroom, or to stop your urine stream when interrupted by a ringing telephone or crying child.

In order to benefit from the exercises, you must be motivated (set aside time *every day*) and patient (the exercises may take 2–3 months to improve your condition). In the beginning, it is best to do the exercises while lying down. You will squeeze the muscle as if trying to hold in rectal gas or pulling the vagina up into your body. If you are not sure, wash your hands and place the first and second fingers of one hand into the vagina. You should feel a squeeze around your fingers. You may also feel as if the fingers are being pulled up into the vagina and forward toward your pubic bone. These are the signs of a proper contraction of this muscle. Avoid contracting your stomach, bottom or leg muscles.

As you progress with the exercise program and both you and the doctor are confident you are doing them properly, you may do the exercises while sitting or standing (a perfect way to pass the time on the subway or bus!). You may also perform this exercise just before a cough or sneeze, climbing stairs, changing position, laughing or lifting something heavy as a way to prevent urine loss (incontinence). These exercises will become a part of your daily life. As with any other exercise, if you don't do them, they don't work.

The Exercises

"Quick Flick"
    Tighten and relax the muscle as quickly as possible 10–20 times in a row. Relax for a count of 10, then repeat. Do _____ repetitions of this exercise, increasing by 5 repetitions each week up to a maximum of 50 repetitions.

"Slow Contraction"
    Tighten the muscle as hard as you can for a count of 10–20. Relax for a count of 10, then repeat. Do _____ repetitions of this exercise, increasing by 5 repetitions each week up to a maximum of 50 repetitions.

"Sustained Contraction"
    Tighten the muscle "halfway" (half as hard as you did for the slow contraction) and hold it for 60 seconds. Relax for a count of 20, then repeat. Do _____ repetitions of this exercise, increasing by 2 repetitions each week up to a maximum of 10 repetitions.

cure rate with the remaining 16% improved utilizing the same 20-min three times daily regimen.[8] He stressed the need for weekly office follow-up and noted distinct phases in the patient education process. The first phase is one of muscle education during which the patient gains awareness and coordination of the pelvic floor with minimal gains in actual muscle strength, followed by a phase of progressive resistive exercise during which the patient strengthens this area as documented by increasing pressures generated on the perineometer. He again stressed the need for frequent office evaluation of progress, additionally stating, "Initial results of this therapeutic plan are so encouraging that examination for function of the pelvic muscles is recommended as a routine procedure in all obstetrical and gynecologic patients." In later work, Kegel reduced utilization of the perineometer only to those women with poor voluntary pelvic floor control and noted 89% overall success within 6 months of therapy in a series of 101 women, some of whom did and others of whom did not use the perineometer during the exercise regimen.[9]

Current Applications

Subsequent studies have shown cure/improvement rates ranging from 50% to 80%. Patient satisfaction is high among those motivated to undertake the therapy.[10] A variety of authors have looked at demographic and clinical factors in an attempt to predict who may be more or less likely to benefit from PFE. Mouritsen et al. found no outcome correlation with patient weight, age, severity of incontinence, or urodynamic diagnosis; however women with a positive estrogen status were 5 times more likely to be cured than those who were hypoestrogenic.[11] Henalla et al. found no correlation with age or severity of stress incontinence but did find improvement to correlate with a shorter duration of incontinence symptoms.[12] Worth et al. found no correlation with age, race, parity, history of episiotomy, or history of prior PFE.[5] McIntosh et al. found no correlation with age, race, weight, parity, or menopause status.[4] Elia and Bergman found that PFE were more likely to improve the incontinence status of women with mild stress urinary incontinence and/or an abdominal/urethral pressure transmission ratio of $\geq$ 80%.[13] Bo et al. found that stress incontinent patients in a supervised PFE group who responded well to PFE were older, more incontinent as per pad test and subjective report, had a longer history of incontinence, weighed more, had stronger pretherapy pelvic floor muscles, negative closure pressure, and lower resting maximum urethral pressure on urodynamics, and were more motivated for treatment than borderline responders.[14] Given that the most significant variables appear to be physician and patient motivation and follow-up, it appears reasonable to encourage any interested patient to try PFE.

Adjunctive Modification

Biofeedback is often used concomitant with PFE in an effort to maximize treatment outcome. Biofeedback involves any process of furnishing an individual information, usually auditory or visual, on the state of one or more physiologic variables, thereby enabling the individual to gain voluntary control over the physiologic variable being sampled. The concept of enhancing PFE efforts is not a new one. Originally, Kegel treated all PFE patients with a form of biofeedback, the perineometer. Given that this device will record pressure increases due to incorrect maneuvers (Valsalva effort) in addition to proper pelvic floor contraction, it is no longer widely utilized. Other methods, in the form of commercial or individually crafted vaginal and rectal pressure balloons, vaginal and rectal probe electromyography (EMG), and concentric needle EMG units are used today (Fig. 4.3).

The utility of concomitant biofeedback has been demonstrated by Burgio et al. in a series of 24 stress incontinent women.[15] Completing a series of four biweekly training sessions, half of the patients were able to see and hear biofeedback from a rectal pressure transducer and the other half were coached with digital palpation by a physiotherapist only. Biofeedback patients documented a 76% decrease in incontinent episodes on diary while those without biofeedback showed a 51% decrease. At 6 months follow-up, similar results were obtained. Susset et al. have also demonstrated an increased clinical response in stress incontinent women with low urethral resistance utilizing PFE and a portable air-filled vaginal probe home biofeedback device.[16] Patients exercised with the probe in place 20 min twice daily. After 6 weeks, there was an 80% subjective cure rate, 87% negative

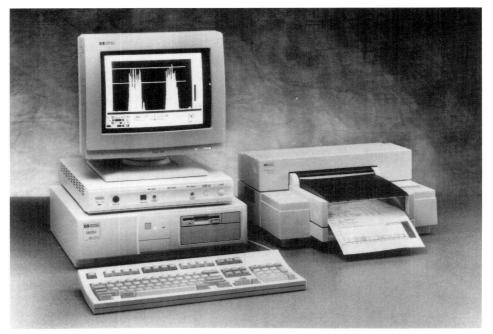

A

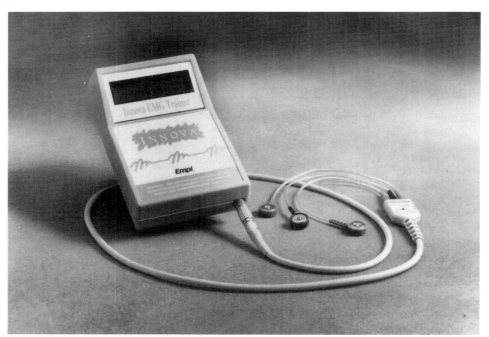

B

Fig. 4.3. A: EMG biofeedback office system. Biofeedback sessions are both audible and visible to the patient. Data can be stored and printed. (Distributed by Empi, Inc.; 800-445-9834). **B:** EMG biofeedback home trainer. Biofeedback can be used daily by the patient to enhance pelvic floor exercise therapy. (Distributed by Empi, Inc., 800-445-9834).

pad test, and a 3–14 fold increase in intravaginal pressure generated on pelvic floor contraction; however only 4 of the 15 women demonstrated an increase in urethral closure pressure. McIntosh et al. utilized pelvic floor exercises with vaginal probe EMG biofeedback and documented improvement in 66% of stress incontinent women, 33% of women with detrusor instability, and 50% of mixed incontinent women, with fecal incontinence reduced in 63% of those reporting this as a concomitant problem.[4]

Burns et al. undertook a randomized, controlled study of 135 older women with stress or mixed incontinence and evaluated the efficacy of pelvic floor exercises both with and without vaginal probe EMG biofeedback versus nontreated controls. They also reported a significant enhancement of therapy when biofeedback was utilized in this older group.[17]

Another, less elaborate, method of biofeedback are weighted vaginal cones (Fig. 4.4). The cones are commercially available in this country in a set of five. They are all identical in dimensions, but vary in weight. The standard regimen involves utilizing the heaviest cone that can be retained for 1 min of ambulation. This cone is then placed in the vagina for 15 min twice daily. We advise patients to test the next heaviest cone on a weekly basis, and to change when it too can be retained for 1 min of ambulation. The biofeedback element exists in the fact that the only way to retain the cone is by proper pelvic floor contraction, and that Valsalva maneuvers will lead to expulsion. The cones are portable and easy to maintain. In a 1-month vaginal cone exercise regimen done by 30 stress inconti-

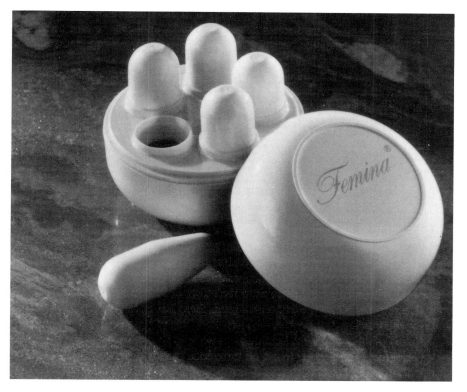

Fig. 4.4. Weighted vaginal cones for pelvic floor rehabilitation. The cones vary in weight and are retained by contracting the pelvic floor. (Distributed by Dacomed, 800-235-1959).

nent women awaiting surgery, 70% were either cured or improved to the extent that only 37% actually went on to have the planned surgical procedure.[18]

Therapeutic Outcome

How long do the results of pelvic floor exercise programs last, and what sort of maintenance regimen is necessary? In one of the largest series (170 stress incontinent women) with long-term follow-up in which a course of physiotherapist-supervised pelvic floor exercises done 4–6 times daily (average 5 months) was employed, Hahn et al. found an initial post-treatment cure rate of 23%, with 48% improved and the remainder unchanged.[3] On follow-up (2–7 years after training completed) via questionnaire, 25% had subsequently elected surgical therapy, with 42% subjectively cured, 21% improved, and 4% unchanged by the operation. Of the nonoperated patients, 11% were subjectively cured, 44% improved, 31% unchanged, and 14% worse. The authors noted that the patients who went on to have surgery had more severe incontinence both subjectively and on pad test prior to beginning the exercise program, and that the likelihood of being cured or improved increased with the length of initial therapy. However, on follow-up, there did not appear to be a correlation between frequency of long-term exercise and self-reported cure or improvement. In a 5 year follow-up of 48 women, a 54% cure/improve rate was present after therapy, with a 58% cure/improve rate found 5 years later among those who had not subsequently undergone surgery.[10] These women had undergone 10 weeks of exercise monitored by a physiotherapist biweekly with daily home exercises "as frequently as possible according to the patient's ability and using it in daily activities." Similar to Hahn's study, 27% had subsequently elected surgery due to incontinence and/or prolapse. And again, there was no correlation between long-term effect and self-reported frequency of home practicing. These data lend support to the concept of acceptable long-term improvement with pelvic floor exercise, and that for motivated patients preferring a nonoperative method, they may expect reasonable results.

The frequency of home exercise in these studies tends to vary, ranging from one session every other day to 6 times daily.[3,19] An average of 20-min sessions 2–3 times daily for 3–6 months is a common regimen. Reasonable post-therapy maintenance regimens and follow-up schedules have not been tested. Patients at our institution are instructed that there is no "end-point" for exercise therapy; as with any other exercise program, one can expect a deterioration if exercises are abandoned. We advise a maintenance schedule of 20 min daily, or at minimum, every other day, with office follow-up every 3–4 months at which time a subjective and pelvic muscle rating scale evaluation are obtained.

The vast majority of research with pelvic floor exercises has been done on stress incontinent women. There have been few studies documenting improvement in adults with detrusor instability.[4,11,17] Pelvic floor exercises have also been used to successfully treat both urge incontinence and discoordinate voiding in children.[20,21]

There is also a dearth of evidence as to the utility of PFE in the treatment of continent women. Despite Dr. Kegel's early enthusiasm, there has been little done in the way of identifying and treating continent women who may benefit from PFE. In a preliminary randomized study of 24 continent nulliparous women with no clinical evidence of pelvic floor disorder or defect, Thorp et al. found no difference in pelvic floor strength in exercisers versus nonexercising controls.[22] Exercisers received detailed instruction at the first visit and performed the exercises 3 times daily for 6 weeks. Controls were not instructed in PFE and also returned in 6 weeks for evaluation. Both digital scale and anal/vaginal EMG recordings showed no significant change in either group. However, given that evidence of stress incontinence has been documented to occur with surprising frequency even among healthy nulliparous women, including college athletes, we can expect further research directed to the utility of PFE for women of all age groups and continence categories.[23,24]

BIOFEEDBACK

While frequently used as an adjunct to pelvic floor exercises, biofeedback has also found utility as primary therapy for detrusor instability with its resultant urgency/frequency and urge incontinence symptoms. In one of the earliest series, Wear et al. used biofeedback to treat a small group of eight men and women with pelvic pain, urinary incontinence, and/or retention.[25] Cystometrics was utilized to provide visible biofeedback and the patients were coached during the sessions with a focus on developing voluntary control of their peri-urethral musculature. Half of the patients noted significant reduction in symptoms, and further studies of biofeedback and bladder dysfunction followed. In a subsequent series of 27 women with detrusor instability, Cardozo et al. undertook a program of biofeedback bladder reeducation carried out during cystometrics.[26] Participants underwent hour-long cystometric sessions at weekly intervals for 4–8 weeks in which an audible and visible biofeedback unit registered increases in bladder pressure. Eighty-two percent of patients reported subjective cure or improvement, while cystometrogram showed a 46% decrease in the provocation of involuntary detrusor contractions and a 52% reduction in demonstrable urge incontinence. While a 5 year follow-up of these women did not document a high rate of persistent therapeutic effect among those initially cured or improved, the authors felt that it remained "worth trying in a highly motivated group of women with a mild to moderate detrusor instability and a good insight into their bladder problems."[27] As with pelvic floor exercises, one might anticipate a dissipation of therapeutic effect in the absence of a maintenance program, and further research in this area is needed. Cystometric biofeedback has also been used with and without adjunctive PFE in the treatment of childhood bladder dysfunction.[21,28,29]

ELECTRICAL STIMULATION

Electric stimulation as a treatment modality for incontinence has been available for over 20 years. It has been demonstrated to be of benefit as primary treatment for stress and urge incontinence, as an adjunctive augmentation to pelvic floor exercise programs and as a method to facilitate proprioception of pelvic floor contraction in biofeedback therapies.

Innervation

This therapy involves the manipulation of bladder and pelvic floor innervation, which is three fold. Storage is effected via the *sympathetic* hypogastric complex originating from T11–L2 which maintains the detrusor in a relaxed state of β-adrenergic stimulation while providing concomitant α-adrenergic stimulation of the internal urethral sphincter, resulting in competent vesical neck contraction. As the bladder fills and approaches capacity, stretch receptors in the bladder wall begin to transmit afferent signals via the *parasympathetic* pelvic nerves (S2,3,4) to the dorsolateral white matter of the spinal cord. Impulses then ascend to the somatosensory area of the cerebral cortex, eliciting sensations of fullness and urgency, and to Barrington's micturition center in the pons. Barrington's center is believed to coordinate bladder and internal urethral sphincter activity during voiding via descending efferent stimulation of the pelvic nerves, with resultant micturition. The third component of innervation involves the *somatic* pudendal nerves, also originating from S2,3,4. Intact somatic innervation allows for voluntary control of the pelvic floor, or levator muscle complex, which, when contracted, functions as an external urethral closure mechanism.

Nerve fiber function varies with size such that the conduction speed increases with fiber width, or diameter and degree of myelination. Group A fibers are the largest and thickly myelinated, involved in motor function and sensory (touch, pressure, temperature) perception. Group B fibers are minimally myelinated, of moderate diameter and are found in the autonomic system, serving visceral organs in a motor and sensory capacity. Group C fibers are unmyelinated, transmit current at the slowest speed, and function primarily in somatic pain reflex responses. Nerve stimulation depends not only on these parameters, but also the proximity of the electrode to the nerve. Various types of electrodes have been utilized, including anal or vaginal probe mounted band electrodes, implanted cuff or wire electrodes, and cutaneous surface electrodes to provide retrograde stimulation of the pudendal nerve and pudendal/pelvic nerve reflex arc, as well as antegrade sacral anterior root stimulation.

Fundamentals of Electricity

Ohm's law (Current = Voltage/Resistance) describes the flow of electrons (current), as a function of the relationship between the force that makes charged particles move (voltage), and capacity of the substance to which current is being applied to store charge and resist opposition to the movement of charged particles (resistance). When applied to the human body, resistance is a property of the tissue adjacent to the electrode, and voltage and current can be varied via the delivery system. In order to reduce the potential for thermal injury, voltage is fixed and current adjustable in most commercially available biomedical stimulation devices (Fig. 4.5). Current to the pelvic floor is delivered in a series of interrupted pulses, usually in a bidirectional (biphasic) waveform. The number of pulses per second is called the frequency, denoted by Hertz (Hz), where one pulse per second = one Hz. The striate muscle of the pelvic floor requires a high stimulation frequency in the range of 20–50+ Hz to effect urethral closure, whereas the bladder inhibition reflex system responds at a lower frequency, with maximal inhibition seen at frequencies of 5–10 Hz.

History

Electric stimulation for the treatment of incontinence was first described by Caldwell in 1963 in the "Preliminary Communications" section of the *Lancet*.[30] Using implanted electrodes attached to a radiofrequency generator, two women, one with a 23-year history of fecal incontinence and the other with a 20-year history of urinary urge incontinence, were cured.

In 1977, Fall and colleagues conducted an elegant series of feline and human studies, elucidating the physiologic mechanisms of action and optimal therapeutic frequency parameters of electrical stimulation of the bladder. In parts I and II, it was determined that intravaginal stimulation accomplished closure of the feline urethra and inhibition of detru-

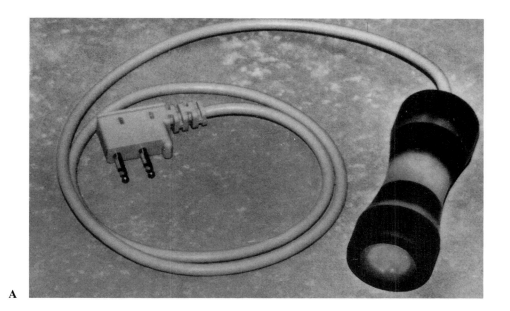

A

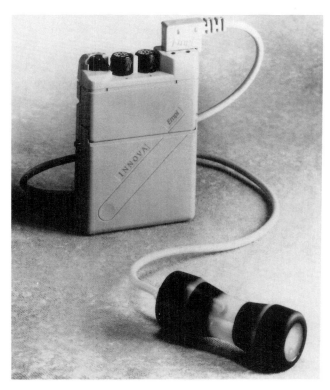

B

Fig. 4.5. A: Vaginal electrode for intravaginal electric stimulation. These carbon band electrodes set in a silicone rubber probe are dual-channel, allowing for stimulation at either 50 Hz (inner bands) or 12.5 Hz (outer bands). (Distributed by Empi, Inc., 800-445-9834). **B:** Portable pelvic floor electric stimulation device with vaginal probe electrode. Patients may undergo daily therapy at home, returning to the office setting for evaluation of progress and adjustment of stimulation parameters. (Distributed by Empi, Inc., 800-445-9834).

sor activity and that these responses could be elicited independent of each other.[31,32] In the remaining studies, carried out with human female volunteers, it was determined that urethral closure was maximal at frequencies of 20–50 Hz (part III) and bladder inhibition best effected at 10 Hz (part IV).[33,34] In part V, differences in response to conduction and general anesthesia were observed, such that a role for electric stimulation in patients with lower motor neuron lesions was proposed.[35] In the final segment (part VI) of this series, a prototype of a commercially available intravaginal stimulation device was successfully tested in women with stress, urge, and mixed incontinence.[36] It was noted that stress incontinence required 4 to 9 months of therapy to effect significant clinical improvement, whereas all urge incontinent patients noted significant improvement within 3 months of treatment.

Chronic Electrical Stimulation Therapy

The earlier studies utilizing anal or vaginal probe mounted electrodes involved long-term treatment protocols. Patients underwent daily stimulation ranging from 6 to 24 hr daily, for anywhere from 1 to 36 months.[36–44] Studies were carried out almost exclusively with participants suffering stress, urge, and mixed incontinence; a few trials included patients with neurogenic bladder dysfunction.[37–39,44,45] Cure, improvement, and failure rates covered a wide range (Fig. 4.6), with those suffering detrusor instability demonstrating a greater likelihood to respond to therapy than those with stress incontinence. Follow-up ranged from 1 month to several years, with no long-term reports documenting the degree to which the therapeutic outcome is persistent.

Maximal Electrical Stimulation Therapy

In one of the earliest studies utilizing short-term, or maximal electric stimulation (MES), Plevnik and Janez treated 98 men and women with stress, urge, and neurogenic incontinence using anal or vaginal probe mounted electrodes.[46] The regimen involved 1–3 treatment sessions lasting only 15–20 min and the results were encouraging, with three mixed incontinence patients remaining cured at 1 year following only one treatment session. The authors proposed that MES appeared to be more efficient and simpler to apply in many

Cure: (0–88%)
Stress Incontinence: 0–78%
Urge Incontinence: 45–89%
Mixed Incontinence: 30–100%

Improved: (6–62%)
Stress Incontinence: 22–78%
Urge incontinence: 11–21%
Mixed Incontinence: 6–35%

Failed: (0–67%)
Stress Incontinence: 0–80%
Urge Incontinence: 0–13%
Mixed Incontinence: 0–12%

Fig. 4.6. Chronic Electric Stimulation Therapy of Stress, Urge and Mixed Incontinence

types of urinary incontinence, as compared to chronic (long-term) stimulation. Some 10 years later, Eriksen et al. utilized weekly or biweekly MES sessions to treat 48 women with detrusor instability, noting an 85% cure/improved rate just after therapy and 77% at one year follow-up.[47] As with long-term therapy, the majority of MES studies have been done with stress, urge, or mixed incontinence patients, using anal and/or vaginal mounted electrodes.

Regimens have ranged from 15- to 20-min sessions carried out anywhere from twice daily to once weekly, with a total number of sessions ranging from 1 to 84. On review of the literature, no regimen appears optimal. For instance, Bent et al. treated a group of stress and urge incontinent women for 15 min twice daily for 6 weeks.[48] At 6 week follow-up, they reported comparable cure/improvement rates for stress (9%/78%) and urge (8%/61%) incontinent patients. Ohlsson et al. treated patients with idiopathic detrusor instability or uninhibited overactive bladder in a series of 4 weekly 20-min sessions, and at 10 months follow-up, found 40% of the idiopathic and 53% of the uninhibited patients to be cured.[49] Caputo et al. treated stress, urge, and mixed incontinent patients in a series of 6 weekly 15-min sessions, reporting cure/improvement in 80% of stress, 63% of urge, and 67% of mixed incontinence patients on follow-up ranging from 2 to 12 months.[50] Additionally, 58% of surgical candidates opted to forgo surgery after completing MES therapy. Schiotz treated stress incontinent women for 20 min per day over a 1-month period, resulting in 12% cure, 33% improvement, 65% failure, and one-third of patients electing to forgo surgical treatment.[51] In a recent multicenter placebo-controlled trial of stress incontinent women, Sand et al. noted a 62% cure/improved rate after 12 weeks of 30-min sessions of intravaginal stimulation performed twice daily.[52] As with chronic electric stimulation therapy, response rates for stress, urge, and mixed incontinence vary greatly with MES (Fig. 4.7) and further study is necessary to evaluate optimization of therapeutic regimens for various categories of incontinence and bladder dysfunction.[46–56]

MES has also been used to treat neurogenic bladder with response rates ranging from 75% cured to 20% increase in the number of incontinent episodes.[45,46,53,54] Sensory urgency (interstitial cystitis) has also been shown to respond, with two studies showing cure rates of 38% and 53%.[53,55] Childhood enuresis resulted in cure/improvement rates of 36%/43% after 1 month of daily MES sessions.[56] Further research application in these areas is needed, as the initial results have all been promising.

Cure: (12–70%)
Stress Incontinence: 9–35%
Urge Incontinence: 8–65%
Mixed Incontinence: N/A

Improved: (32–76%)
Stress Incontinence: 33–89%
Urge Incontinence: 30–63%
Mixed Incontinence: 67%

Failed: (17–65%)
Stress Incontinence: 13–65%
Urge Incontinence: 5–37%
Mixed Incontinence: 33%

Fig. 4.7. Maximal Electric Stimulation Therapy of Stress, Urge and Mixed Incontinence

Interferential Therapy

Interferential electric stimulation (IFT) another method of delivering current to the pelvic floor, utilizes either two or four external patch or suction cup electrodes. The electrodes are placed such that stimulation results in two perpendicular high-frequency (2–4 kHz) currents which cross, or "interfere," at the level of the pelvic floor. Despite these high frequencies, due to increased current impedance across the area of the pelvis, perceptible stimulation occurs only in the area of interference. The currents are set at slightly different intensities, and this difference becomes the low-frequency therapeutic interferential current (i.e., a 10-Hz difference becomes a 10-Hz pelvic floor stimulation).

The advantage to interferential therapy is the lack of invasiveness; no devices are placed within the vagina or rectum and no needles are implanted. It is a method routinely used by many pelvic floor physiotherapists, almost exclusively outside of the U.S.[57–60] The most common electrode placement involves two electrodes above the inguinal ligament and two applied to the inner thigh near the groin. Using an intravaginal pressure sensor, Green and Laycock demonstrated that this was the least effective method, with greatest pelvic floor contractions demonstrated when two electrodes were placed just lateral and anterior to the anus.[57] In a comparison of weighted vaginal cones to IFT, Olah et al. demonstrated no significant difference in subjective or objective improvement between the two groups, however the cup electrodes were placed in the standard (2 inguinal, 2 adductor), and possibly least effective, position.[58] In a comparison of PFE with and without adjunctive IFT, Wilson et al. showed significant increases in vaginal pressure in the PFE/IFT group with no improvement in the PFE-only group.[59] However, in a comparison of PFE, IFT and local premarin creme, PFE alone resulted in 65% improvement, as opposed to IFT alone (32%) and local estrogen creme alone (12%).[60] Thus, while encouraging when considering patient comfort and compliance, there is no consensus as to the efficacy of IFT at this time.

Transcutaneous Electric Nerve Stimulation

Transcutaneous electric nerve stimulation (TENS) applied suprapubically has been demonstrated to successfully treat both ulcerative and nonulcerative interstitial cystitis.[61] The acupuncture points for the bladder are located over the peroneal (L5) and posterior tibial (S1) nerves and have been shown to successfully treat detrusor instability.[62,63] These results generated interest in the possibility of enhancing the response with electrical stimulation, and TENS therapy of the posterior tibial nerve has been tried in patients with detrusor instability, neurogenic bladder, and/or interstitial cystitis with both encouraging and discouraging results.[64,65]

Sacral Anterior Root Stimulation

Manipulation of bladder storage and emptying functions via direct neural stimulation has been under investigation for over 25 years.[66–69] This form of electric stimulation therapy involves application of electrodes such that they are imbedded, lying in direct contact with the anterior sacral roots. Efferent stimulation of the nerve roots then effects contraction of the striate sphincter and levator musculature via the somatic pudendal fibers. Micturition is effected by a phenomenon known as *post-stimulation voiding,* wherein the parasympathetic pelvic nerves, also activated by sacral root stimulation via the sacral reflex arc, continue to fire after stimulation has stopped and the external sphincter/pelvic floor relaxed, effecting a detrusor contraction/bladder evacuation. In patients with detrusor hyperreflexia, reflex detrusor contractions can be abolished by concomitant posterior root rhizotomy.

In a series of canine studies, optimal stimulation parameters for sphincteric closure were demonstrated at a frequency of 20 Hz with a duty cycle (on:off time) of 50 milliseconds:100 milliseconds.[70] On histochemical study of the striate urethral sphincter, hypertrophy and increased glycolytic activity (denoting increased fatigue resistance) were demonstrated after stimulation. Nerve damage can be minimized by stimulating at a frequency of 15–20 Hz at amplitudes of less than 4 milliamps.

General anesthesia and dissection of the sacral foramina allows exact implantation. Intraoperative urodynamics and concomitant electrostimulation can be utilized to identify the sacral roots responsible for micturition. The anterior and posterior roots are then identified, and if indicated, selective posterior rhizotomy can also be performed. The leads are tunneled under the skin to the anterior abdominal wall where it is connected to an imbedded stimulator to facilitate easy access and control by the patient.[71] Other investigators have hooked the cables to a subcutaneous radio receiver which is then in turn activated by an external radiotransmitter.[72]

Current patient selection requires history of failure of conventional therapeutic methods, intact sacral motor neurons (i.e., pelvic nerves which are capable of responding to direct sacral stimulation via the sacral reflex arc), and a functional detrusor. The stimulation sessions are frequently painful, and patients with intact or partial sensory function should undergo pain tolerance testing prior to permanent implantation.

In the neurogenic patient, posterior root rhizotomy is often performed at the time of implantation in order to maximize the goals of inhibiting detrusor hyperreflexia and permitting complete and reliable electromicturition. Posterior root rhizotomy results in loss of sensory input at and below the level of ablation, and therefore is avoided in neurologically intact patients. Patients with incomplete cord lesions and intact sensory function need to be carefully counseled regarding the benefits of the combined procedure (continence, adequate bladder compliance, and absence of detrusor-sphincter dyssynergia) versus the risk of further impairment of S2–5 sensation with loss of reflex erections and vaginal dryness being common complications.[72,73]

In long-term follow-up, it has demonstrated the greatest efficacy in patients with "an element of detrusor hyperreflexia who retain a moderate degree of sphincteric function and external sphincteric responsiveness to neural stimulation."[71] However, application in neurologically intact urge incontinent and postprostatectomy sphincteric incontinence has been successful as well.[71] A role for anterior root stimulation in the treatment of neurogenic defecation disorders has also been demonstrated.[74]

BEHAVIORAL THERAPY

Behavioral therapy involves systematic manipulation of environmental and behavioral variables related to the specific dysfunction; when applied to the bladder, operant conditioning and systematic desensitization are most commonly employed. Also called bladder training, habit training, bladder drill, and bladder reeducation, behavioral therapy has been utilized to treat urge syndromes, interstitial cystitis, and urinary incontinence in the elderly.

Urge Syndromes

In treating urge syndromes/detrusor instability, daily voiding diaries in which the patient records the time and volume of each void and incontinent episodes are most commonly involved. The intervoiding interval is increased weekly by 15–30 min until the desired intervoiding interval (3–4 h) is obtained. It has frequently been combined with short-term anticholinergic drug therapy which is gradually withdrawn after bladder function is normalized.[75–77] In one of the earliest series, Frewen treated 50 detrusor instability patients with 10 days of in-house bladder training, adjunctive short-term pharmacotherapy and monthly outpatient follow-up.[75] Results were encouraging with an 82% short-term cure rate which was maintained (80%) at 1 year follow-up. However, in a comparison of bladder drill alone with standard drug therapy, Jarvis found a post-treatment continence rate of 84% in bladder drill patients versus 56% in the drug therapy group at 3 months follow-up.[78] Despite these findings, anticholinergic therapy remains the first treatment choice of most gynecologists and urologists for the treatment of detrusor instability.

In order to ascertain whether or not response to therapy varies with urodynamic diagnosis, Holmes et al. evaluated 56 patients with urge syndrome and categorized them into detrusor instability, urge symptoms without cystometric detrusor instability, and urge syndrome due to decreased bladder compliance.[77] All participants undertook identical programs of bladder training; anticholinergic therapy was used initially and withdrawn at 3 months. Initial overall cure/improvement rate was 85%. However, at 1–5 years follow-up, differences in therapeutic persistence became evident. The patients without demonstrable detrusor instability and normal compliance maintained a high level of relief, but patients with urodynamically demonstrated detrusor instability and/or decreased bladder compliance had a relapse rate of 43%. Conversely, Mahady and Begg treated 48 patients, all with cystometric evidence of detrusor instability, with behavioral therapy, short-term pharmacotherapy, and adjunctive psychotherapy.[76] At 4 years follow-up, a 90% subjective cure rate and 77% cystometric detrusor stability was found.

Interstitial Cystitis

Interstitial cystitis, or sensory urgency, has also been successfully treated with behavioral therapy.[79,80] One of the salient clinical components of this most troubling disorder is that the patient suffers constant sensations of bladder fullness or pressure even when empty, with severe urgency suffered at low volumes, often less than 50–100 ml, leading to the classic complaint of "living life in the bathroom" with minimal relief between voids. Ignoring all potential micropathophysiologic explanations, behavioral therapy in this group focuses on desensitization, literally a "potty training," so that the patient senses initial bladder fullness and intense bladder urgency only at normal volumes. Technique is similar to that of detrusor instability protocols, with the patient keeping a daily bladder diary, maintaining a set intervoiding interval, which is increased at weekly intervals. Adjunctive PFE has also been utilized to reduce sensations of urgency and, conversely, to aid in reduction of the confounding discoordinate voiding which so often accompanies this syndrome.[79]

Using an inpatient bladder drill protocol only, Jarvis demonstrated a 60% cure rate at 6 months follow-up.[80] In a 3-month outpatient treatment series of timed void diaries, fluid intake manipulation, and adjunctive PFE, Chaikin et al. demonstrated 88% success in a group of 42 women with refractory interstitial cystitis.[79] This type of therapy is labor-intensive for both patient and physician or therapist, requiring a high level of motivation and frequent follow-up in the outpatient setting.

Elder Incontinence

Various categories of behavioral therapy have found practical application in the reduction of incontinence among the elderly.[81–84] Incontinence in this age group is much more likely to be multifaceted in etiology, with impaired neurologic, mental status and physical mobility and fecal impaction often compounding primary bladder dysfunction such as detrusor instability or intrinsic sphincter incompetence. Voiding diaries can be used to increase intervoiding interval, or to tailor voiding and/or volume intake to documented diurnal variations in incontinence so as to reduce the degree of incontinence. In neurologically impaired patients, a set schedule of spontaneous or self-catheterized voiding can reduce neurogenic incontinence and protect the upper urinary tract. Cognitively impaired patients may be placed on a set schedule of prompted voiding, in which they are reminded to void at set intervals by family or caretakers. Using adjunctive cystometric biofeedback, Burgio et al. demonstrated an 82–94% reduction in incontinent episodes among a group of elderly stress and urge incontinent outpatients.[81] Utility among institutional elderly has also been demonstrated.[82,83]

CONCLUSION

Pelvic floor exercise, biofeedback, electrical stimulation, and behavior modification therapies have been effective individually and in various combinations for the treatment of a wide variety of bladder disorders. Optimal patient care entails individual tailoring, and not all clinical candidates will be willing or able to comply with established treatment regimens, preferring surgery or pharmacotherapy as first-line measures. However, for those interested and capable, they may expect a reasonable degree of relief in over half of those so treated. Long-term follow-up is needed so that the appropriate comparisons to surgical methods can be made. Additionally, maintenance regimens may be in order for patients treated with these methods, and work in this area is also needed.

It is most important to remind patients that a suboptimal response to the therapies listed here does not necessarily mean that they "didn't do it correctly." As when treating any other chronic condition with its inevitable toll on lifestyle and self-perception, encouragement, close follow-up, and flexibility can be as important to a successful treatment as any individual therapeutic method.

REFERENCES

1. Bump RC, Hurt WG, Fantl JA, et al: Assessment of Kegel pelvic muscle exercise performance after brief verbal instruction. *Am J Obstet Gynecol* 165:322–329, 1991.

2. Bo K, Hagen RH, Kvarstein B, et al: Pelvic floor muscle exercise for the treatment of female stress urinary incontinence: III. Effects of two different degrees of pelvic floor muscle exercises. *Neurourol Urodyn* 9:489–502, 1990.

3. Hahn I, Milsom I, Fall M, et al: Long-term results of pelvic floor training in female stress urinary incontinence. *Br J Urol* 72:421–427, 1993.

4. McIntosh LJ, Frahm JD, Mallett VT, et al: Pelvic floor rehabilitation in the treatment of incontinence. *J Repro Med* 38:662–666, 1993.

5. Worth AM, Dougherty MC, McKey PL: Development and testing of the circumvaginal muscles rating scale. *Nurs Res* 35:166–168, 1986.

6. Brink CA, Wells TJ, Sampselle CM, et al: A digital test for pelvic muscle strength in women with urinary incontinence. *Nurs Res* 43:352–356, 1994.

7. Kegel AH: Progressive resistance exercise in the functional restoration of the perineal muscles. *Am J Obstet Gynecol* 56:238–248, 1948.

8. Kegel AH: Physiologic therapy for urinary stress incontinence. *JAMA* July:915–917, 1951.

9. Jones EG, Kegel AH: Treatment of urinary stress incontinence. *Surg Gynec Obstet* 94:179–189, 1952.

10. Cammu H, Van Nylen M: Pelvic floor muscle exercises: 5 years later. *Urology* 45:113–118, 1995.

11. Mouritsen L, Frimodt-Moller C, Moller M: Long-term effect of pelvic floor exercises on female urinary incontinence. *Br J Urol* 68:32–37, 1991.

12. Henalla SM, Sirwan P, Castleden CM, et al: The effect of pelvic floor exercises in the treatment of genuine urinary stress incontinence in women at two hospitals. *Br J Obstet Gynaecol* 95:602–606, 1988.

13. Elia G, Bergman A: Pelvic muscle exercises: when do they work? *Obstet Gynecol* 81:283–286, 1993.

14. Bo K, Larsen S: Pelvic floor muscle exercise for the treatment of female stress urinary incontinence: classification and characterization of responders: *Neurourol Urodyn* 11:497–507, 1992.

15. Burgio KL, Robinson JC, Engel BT: The role of biofeedback in Kegel exercise training for stress urinary incontinence. *Am J Obstet Gynecol* 154:58–64, 1986.

16. Susset JG, Galea G, Read L: Biofeedback therapy for female incontinence due to low urethral resistance. *J Urol* 143:1205–1208, 1990.

17. Burns PA, Pranikoff K, Nochajski TH, et al: A comparison of effectiveness of biofeedback and pelvic muscle exercise treatment of stress incontinence in older community-dwelling women. *J Gerontol* 48:M167–M174, 1993.

18. Peattie AB, Plevnik S, Stanton SL: Vaginal cones: a conservative method of treating genuine stress incontinence: *Br J Obstet Gynaecol* 95:1049–1053, 1988.

19. Doughterty M, Bishop K, Mooney R, et al: Graded pelvic muscle exercise effect on stress urinary incontinence. *J Repro Med* 38:684–691, 1993.

20. Schneider MS, King LR, Surwit RS: Kegel exercises and childhood incontinence: a new role for an old treatment. *J Pediatr* 124:91–92, 1994.

21. Kjolseth D, Knudsen KM, Madsen B, et al: Urodynamic biofeedback training for children with bladder-sphincter dyscoordination during voiding. *Neurourol Urodyn* 12:211–212, 1993.

22. Thorp JM, Stephenson H, Jones LH: Pelvic floor (Kegel) exercises—a pilot study in nulliparous women. *Int Urogynecol J* 5:86–89, 1994.

23. Wolin KG: Stress incontinence in young, healthy, nulliparous female subjects. *J Urol* 101:545–549, 1969.

24. Nygaard IE, Thompson FL, Svengalis SL, et al: Urinary incontinence in elite nulliparous athletes. *Obstet Gynecol* 84:183–187, 1994.

25. Wear JB, Wear RB, Cleeland C: Biofeedback in urology using urodynamics: preliminary observations. *J Urol* 121:464–468, 1979.

26. Cardozo LD, Abrams PD, Stanton SL, et al: Idiopathic bladder instability treated by biofeedback. *Br J Urol* 50:521–523, 1978.

27. Cardozo LD, Stanton SL: Biofeedback: a 5-year review. *Br J Urol* 56:220, 1984.

28. Kjolseth DK, Madsen B, Knuden KM, et al: Biofeedback treatment of children and adults with idiopathic detrusor instability. *Scand J Urol Nephrol* 28:243–247, 1994.

29. Sugar E: Bladder control through biofeedback. *Am J Nurs* Aug:1152–1154, 1983.

30. Caldwell KPS: The electrical control of sphincter incompetence. *Lancet* 2:174–175, 1963.

31. Erlandson BE, Fall M, Carlsson CA, et al: The effect of intravaginal electrical stimulation on the feline urethra and urinary bladder. Electrical parameters. *Scand J Urol Nephrol* suppl 44:part I, 1978.

32. Fall M, Erlandson BE, Carlsson CA, et al: The effect of intravaginal electrical stimulation on the feline urethra and urinary bladder. Neuronal mechanisms. *Scand J Urol Nephrol* suppl 44:part II, 1978.

33. Erlandson BE, Magnus F, Sundin T: Intravaginal electrical stimulation. Clinical experiments on urethral closure. *Scand J Urol Nephrol* suppl 44:part III, 1978.

34. Fall M, Erlandson BE, Sundin T, et al: Intravaginal electrical stimulation. Clinical experiments on bladder inhibition. *Scand J Urol Nephrol* suppl 44:part IV, 1978.

35. Erlandson BE, Fall M, Carlsson CA, et al: Mechanisms for closure of the human urethra during intravaginal electrical stimulation. *Scand J Urol Nephrol* suppl 44:part V, 1978.

36. Fall M, Erlandson BE, Nilson AE, et al: Long-term intravaginal electrical stimulation in urge and stress incontinence. *Scand J Urol Nephrol* suppl 44:part VI, 1978.

37. Godec C, Cass AS, Ayala GF: Bladder inhibition with functional electrical stimulaltion. *Urology* 6:663–666, 1975.

38. Godec C, Cass AS, Ayala GF: Electrical stimulation for incontinence. *Urology* 7:388–397, 1976.

39. Sotiropolous A, Yeaw S, Lattimer JK: Management of urinary incontinence with electronic stimulation: observations and results. *J Urol* 116:747–750, 1976.

40. Fall M: Does electrostimulation cure urinary incontinence? *J Urol* 131:664–667, 1984.

41. Fall M, Ahlstrom K, Carlsson CA, et al: Contelle: pelvic floor stimulator for female stress–urge incontinence. *Urology* 28:282–287, 1986.

42. Eriksen BC, Bergmann S, Mjolnerod OK: Effect of anal electrostimulation with the "Incontan" device in women with urinary incontinence. *Br J Obstet Gynaecol* 94:147–156, 1987.

43. Eriksen BC, Mjolnerod OK: Changes in urodynamic measurements after successful anal electrostimulation in female urinary incontinence. *Br J Urol* 59:45–49, 1987.

44. Leach GE, Bavendam TG: Prospective evaluation of the Incontan transrectal stimulator in women with urinary incontinence. *Neurourol Urodynam* 8:231–235, 1989.

45. Ishigooka M, Hashimoto T, Izumiya K, et al: Electrical pelvic floor stimulation in the management of urinary incontinence due to neuropathic overactive bladder. *Front Med Biol Eng* 5:1–10, 1993.

46. Plevnik S, Janez J: Maximal electrical stimulation for urinary incontinence. *Urology* 14:638–646, 1979.

47. Eriksen BC, Bergman S, Eik-Nes SH: *Neurourol Urodynam* 8:219–232, 1989.

48. Bent AE, Sand PK, Ostergard DR: Transvaginal electrostimulation in the therapy of genuine stress incontinence and detrusor instability. *Neurourol Urodynam* 8:363, 1989.

49. Ohlsson BL, Fall M, Frankenberg-Sommar S: Effects of external and direct pudendal nerve maximal electrical stimulation in the treatment of the uninhibited overactive bladder. *Br J Urol* 64:374–380, 1989.

50. Caputo TM, Benson JT, McClellan E: Intravaginal maximal electrical stimulation on the treatment of urinary incontinence. *J Repro Med* 38:667–671, 1993.

51. Schiotz HJ: One month maximal electrostimulation for genuine stress incontinence in women. *Neurourol Urodynam* 13:43–50, 1994.

52. Sand PK, Richardson DA, Staskin DR, et al: Pelvic floor stimulation in the treatment of genuine stress incontinence: a multicenter, placebo-controlled trial. *Proc Symposium Women's Urol Health Res* Mar 1993.

53. Zollner-Nielsen M, Samuelsson SM: Maximal electrical stimulation of patients with frequency, urgency and urge incontinence. *Acta Obstet Gynecol Scand* 71:629–630, 1992.

54. Lamhut P, Jackson TW, Wall LL: The treatment of urinary incontinence with electrical stimulation in nursing home patients: a pilot study. *JAGS* 40:48–52, 1992.

55. Eriksen BC: Painful bladder disease in women: effect of maximal electrical pelvic floor stimulation. *Neurourol Urodynam* 84:362, 1989.

56. Plevnik S, Janez J, Vrtacnik P et al: Short-term electrical stimulation: home treatment for urinary incontinence. *World J Urol* 4:24–26, 1986.

57. Green RJ, Laycock J: Objective methods for evaluation of interferential therapy in the treatment of incontinence. *Transact Biomed Eng* 37:615–623, 1990.

58. Olah KS, Bridges N, Denning J, et al: The conservative management of patients with symptoms of stress incontinence: a randomized, prospective study comparing weighted vaginal cones and interferential therapy. *Am J Obstet Gynecol* 162:87–92, 1990.

59. Wilson PD, Samarrai TA, Deakin M, et al: *Br J Obstet Gynaecol* 94:575–582, 1987.

60. Henalla SM, Hutchins CJ, Robinson P, et al: Non-operative methods in the treatment of female genuine stress incontinence of urine. *J Obstet Gynecol* 9:222–225, 1989.

61: Fall M, Lindstrom S: Transcutaneous electrical nerve stimulation in classical and nonulcer interstitial cystitis. *Urol Clin North Am* 21:131–139, 1994.

62: Pigne A, De Goursac C, Barrat J: Acupuncture and unstable bladder. *Proc 15th Annual Meeting International Continence Society,* London 186–187, 1985.

63: Philip T, Shah PJR, Worth PHL: Acupuncture in the treatment of bladder instability. *Br J Urol* 61:490–493, 1988.

64. McGuire EJ, Shi-Chun Z, Horwinski R, et al: Treatment of motor and sensory detrusor instability by electrical stimulation. *J Urol* 129:78–79, 1983.

65. Geirsson G, Wang YH, Lindstrom S, et al: Traditional acupuncture and electrical stimulation of the posterior tibial nerve. *Scand J Urol Nephrol* 27:67–70, 1993.

66. Ingersoll EJ, Jones LL, Hegre ES: Effect on urinary bladder of unilateral stimulation of pelvic nerves in the dog. *Am J Physiol* 189:167–171, 1957.

67. Holmquist B: Electromicturition by pelvic nerve stimulation in dogs. *Scand J Urol Nephrol* suppl 2:1, 1968.

68. Heine JP, Schmidt RA, Tanagho EA: Intraspinal sacral root stimulation for controlled micturition. *Invest Urol* 15:78–83, 1977.

69. Brindley GS: Emptying the bladder by stimulating sacral ventral roots. *J Physiol* 137:15–16, 1973.

70. Tanagho EA, Schmidt RA: Electrical stimulaltion in the clinical management of the neurogenic bladder. *J Urol* 140:1331–1339, 1988.

71. Tanagho EA: Electrical stimulation. *JAGS* 38:352–355, 1990.

72: Madersbacher H, Fischer J, Ebner A: Anterior sacral root stimulator (Brindley): experiences especially in women with neurogenic urinary incontinence: *Neurourol Urodyn* 7:593–601, 1988.

73: Madersbacher H, Fisher J: Sacral anterior root stimulation: prerequisites and indications. *Neurourol Urodyn* 12:489–494, 1993.

74. Brindley GS, Rushton DN: Long-term follow-up of patients with sacral anterior root stimulator implants. *Paraplegia* 28:569–575, 1990.

75. Frewen W: Role of bladder training in the treatment of the unstable bladder in the female. *Urol Clin North Am* 6:273–277, 1979.

76. Mahady UW, Begg BM: Long-term symptomatic and cystometric cure of the urge incontinence syndrome using a technique of bladder re-education. *Br J Obstet Gynaecol* 88:1038–1043, 1981.

77. Holmes DM, Stone AR, Bary PR, et al: Bladder training—3 years on. *Br J Urol* 55:660–664, 1983.

78. Jarvis GJ: A controlled trial of bladder drill and drug therapy in the management of detrusor instability. *Br J Urol* 53:565–566, 1981.

79. Chaikin DC, Blaivas JG, Blaivas ST: Behavioral therapy for the treatment of refractory interstitial cystitis. *J Urol* 149:1445–1448, 1993.

80. Jarvis GJ: The management of urinary incontinence due to primary vesical sensory urgency by bladder drill. *Br J Urol* 54:374–376, 1982.

81. Burgio KL, Whitehead WE, Engel BT: Urinary incontinence in the elderly. Bladder-sphincter biofeedback and toileting skills training. *Ann Intern Med* 104:507–515, 1985.

82. Ouslander JG, Blaustein J, Connor A, et al: Habit training and oxybutynin for incontinence in nursing home patients: a placebo controlled trial. *JAGS* 36:40–46, 1988.

83. Hu TW, Igou JF, Kaltreider DL, et al: A clinical trial of a behavioral therapy to reduce urinary incontinence in nursing homes. *JAMA* 261:2656–2662, 1989.

84. Hadley EC: Bladder training and related therapies for urinary incontinence in older people. *JAMA* 256:372–379, 1986.

5

Surgery for Stress Incontinence in Women

Jerry G. Blaivas
Dianne M. Heritz

The surgical treatment of stress urinary incontinence has a long and variegated history. The fact that there are over 125 operations described in the literature attests to the notion that no one single procedure has gained widespread acceptance. From a conceptual standpoint, there are six kinds of operations: vaginal urethral plications, transvaginal (needle) bladder neck suspensions, retropubic procedures, pubovaginal sling, prosthetic sphincters, and periurethral injections. The latter two procedures are described in detail in Chapters 6 and 8 and will not be discussed in this section.

INDICATIONS AND CHOICE OF PROCEDURE

The selection of a particular surgical technique is based upon the underlying anatomic and physiologic abnormalities responsible for incontinence, the need for concomitant retropubic or vaginal procedures, the preference and surgical skills of the surgeon, and the expectations of the patient.

When the underlying pathophysiology is urethral hypermobility, the goal of surgery is to prevent the abnormal descent of the vesical neck and proximal urethra. This may be accomplished with any of the vaginal or retropubic suspension operations or by pubovaginal sling. Short-term results are comparable with these procedures; all provide success rates of 80–95%. However, longer term results suggest that pubovaginal sling and the other retropubic operations have a higher success rate than transvaginal bladder neck suspensions or vaginal urethral plications.

Although some surgeons believe that transvaginal bladder neck suspensions and retropubic procedures are effective for some patients with intrinsic sphincter deficiency (ISD),[1–3] we believe that the overall cure rate is no more than about 50% and, therefore, do not recommend these procedures for ISD. The most effective treatment for intrinsic sphincter deficiency is pubovaginal sling.[4–18] Sphincter prosthesis has been advocated by some authors, and in the hands of the experienced prosthetic surgeon the success rate approaches that of pubovaginal sling.[19,20] However, it is difficult for us to justify the additional expense and potential morbidity due to erosion, infection, and mechanical malfunction.

The role of periurethral injection of autologous fat, collagen, Teflon, or silicone particles has not been established. Short-term improvement is seen in most patients with intrinsic sphincter deficiency, but in those with urethral hypermobility, the results have been disappointing. Moreover, repeated injections are almost always necessary and long-term results and complications have not been adequately assessed.[21–24]

In some patients, particularly those who have undergone previous vaginal surgery, there is scarring and fixation of the vesical neck and proximal urethra to the vagina (Type IIB stress urinary incontinence). Surgical treatment in these patients is designed to restore these structures to their normal anatomic position by freeing them of their vaginal attachments, then preventing abnormal descent by any of the foregoing procedures.[25]

Although the need for concomitant surgery should be taken into account when deciding between a vaginal and abdominal approach, one should not compromise the general principles of repair to accommodate another operation. Repair of enterocele and uterine prolapse can be performed either abdominally or vaginally at the same time as the incontinence procedure. Repair of cystocele can be repaired abdominally when there is a paravaginal defect, but central defects must be closed through a vaginal approach. In some patients, rectoceles can also be repaired through the abdomen (provided that concomitant perineorrhaphy is not required), but in most instances a vaginal approach is necessary.

The preferences and skills of the surgeon are of paramount importance in selecting the best surgical approach. It is not enough to select the most appropriate operation for the patient; the surgeon must be skilled and comfortable with the chosen technique. It is far more preferable for the surgeon to continue to perform an operation which has proven successful in his hands than to switch to the latest modification of the newest technique. Too many times we have witnessed the devastating complications that result when an inexperienced surgeon tries out new techniques which hold great promise for improved efficacy with less morbidity. The current emphasis on cost-effectiveness and reduced morbidity is an admirable goal, but one which must be tempered with the reality of good clinical science and the necessity of adequate surgical training.

In our judgment, pubovaginal sling is the most effective and durable operation for urinary incontinence due to either urethral hypermobility or intrinsic sphincter deficiency and we recommend it routinely for both kinds of patients. However, because of the propensity for the inexperienced surgeon to apply too much tension at the time of tying the sling in place, it is not generally recommended as a primary procedure. Another alternative, of course, is for more surgeons to become skilled with this technique!

VAGINAL URETHRAL PLICATION

Howard Kelly first described the plication of periurethral tissues for the treatment of female stress urinary incontinence (Fig. 5.1).[26] His "plication" was intended to correct an open bladder neck which he believed to be the cause of stress urinary incontinence. The

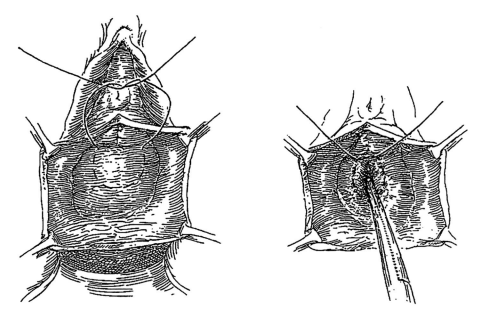

Fig. 5.1. Original Kelly plication. Through a midline vaginal incision, the musculofascial tissue adjacent to the vesical neck is plicated in the midline. It is important that this plication is not done too tightly lest urethral obstruction or devascularization result. (From Nichols and Randall, ref. 26a, with permission.)

popularity of this vaginal procedure became worldwide in Kelly's time and with modification is still performed today.[27] These modifications include elevation of the urethra with plication of endopelvic fascia under the bladder neck and fixation of the fascia to the posterior pubic symphysis[27] (Fig. 5.2). The Kelly plication or anterior repair has a long-term success rate from 35% to 65%. In most comparative studies it is less effective than the other procedures.[28–31] In one randomized control study with 12 month follow-up, comparing Kelly plication, Pereyra and Burch procedures, the success rates were 65%, 72%, and 91% respectively.[32]

TRANSVAGINAL (NEEDLE) VESICAL NECK SUSPENSIONS

Vesical neck suspensions are indicated only in patients with urethral hypermobility. In our judgment, the goal of this surgery is to prevent abnormal descent of the vesical neck and proximal urethra, not to reposition the vesical neck "in a high retropubic position" as some authorities have recommended.[33] In the supine or lithotomy position, with the patient anesthetized, the vesical neck is in the normal anatomic position. It is not necessary, therefore, to apply excess tension on the "suspension sutures." Rather, it is only necessary to remove the slack so that the sutures prevent further descent during increases in abdominal pressure.

We believe that the most common cause of morbidity after incontinence operations is "tying the sutures too tightly." If the sutures are tied too tightly, urethral obstruction ensues

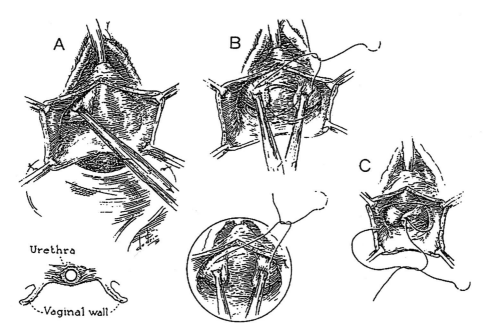

Fig. 5.2. Modified Kelly plication. **A:** The musculofascial supporting structures adjacent to the vesical neck are dissected off the vaginal wall. **B:** The tissue is advanced to the midline and **C:** tied in the midline with an absorbable suture. (From Nichols and Randall, ref. 26a, with permission).

or the patient develops troublesome symptoms of detrusor instability. If they are tied too loosely, there may be no benefit at all. If the suspension sutures are placed too close to the urethra, there is a tendency to cause obstruction or to perforate or erode and cause fistula. If they are placed too far laterally, when the surgeon "pulls up on the sutures" he simply pulls on the attachments of the endopelvic fascia to the bone with no net effect. If the sutures are placed too far proximally there is the possibility of ureteral or bladder injury and if they are placed too far distally, they do not prevent vesical neck descent, and are ineffective in curing incontinence.

Notwithstanding these considerations, the short-term results of needle suspensions consistently show a cure or improvement rate in excess of 80%. Although the data is very incomplete, there is increasing evidence that the long-term cure rate is 50–60%.[34]

In 1959, Pereyra[35] described the needle urethropexy. Through a small vaginal and suprapubic incision, a long needle was passed just behind the symphysis pubis through the retropubic space and lateral to the urethra. The periurethral tissue was transfixed using wire sutures. The needle was then passed on the contralateral side and the two wire sutures tied above in the abdomen "elevating the vesical neck."

The original Pereyra operation has undergone considerable change in the hands of a new generation of surgeons. A number of operations, collectively known as the modified Pereyra procedures have recently gained great popularity. Although the operations seem, at first glance, to be minor modifications of a single procedure, there are important physiologic differences between them. All of these procedures place large, nonabsorbable sutures in the periurethral tissue adjacent to the vesical neck, and transfer the sutures beneath the pubis through the retropubic space and above the rectus fascia. Stamey[36] described a technique using a cystoscopic control and Dacron buttresses over the sutures to prevent them from pulling through the tissues. Cobb and Radge[37] used a double-prong needle to reduce the number of retropubic needle passes, Gittes[38] made no vaginal incision at all. In the Raz[39] modification, the endopelvic fascia is perforated and the retropubic space entered at the lateral attachment of the endopelvic fascia to the pelvic sidewalls. In so doing, the vesical neck and proximal urethra are mobilized. Helical sutures are placed in the endopelvic fascia, the long ends of the sutures are passed to the suprapubic region using a long needle, and the sutures are tied in the midline (Fig. 5.3). In this procedure the strength and integrity of the sutures can be tested and if the tissue appears too weak, other surgical options may be chosen.

The advantages of the Raz operation over the Stamey and Cobb-Radge are entirely technical in nature, but very important. In the latter procedures there is no dissection in the retropubic space and no detachment of the endopelvic fascia from the pelvic sidewalls. Accordingly, there is no way of gauging the distance from the needle insertion to the urethra. If the needle is placed too close to the urethra, obstruction may occur. If it is placed too far laterally, when one pulls up the tissue, it is pulled taut against the bone, but no ele-

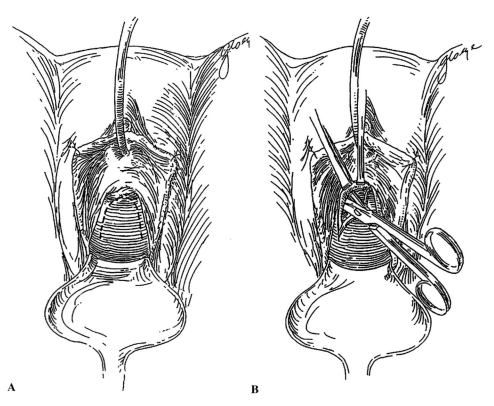

A   **B**

Fig. 5.3. Raz procedure. **A:** An inverted "U" or two oblique incisions are made in the anterior vaginal wall over the vesical neck. **B:** At the level of the vesical neck, a plane is developed just beneath the vaginal epithelium with the tip of the scissors pointed toward the patient's ipsilateral shoulder.

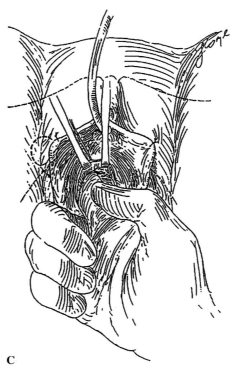

C

C: The retropubic space is entered either with the scissor or the surgeon's index finger at the lateral most margin of the musculofascial tissue.

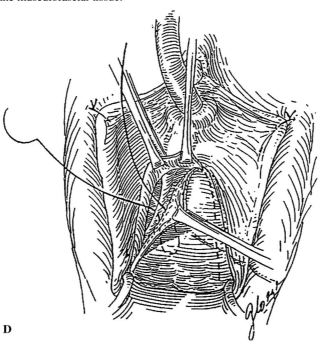

D

D: A number 1 or 2 monofilament nonabsorbable suture is placed in a helical fashion including the entire vaginal wall excluding the epithelium. Alternatively, if a vaginal wall sling is preferred, the first pair of sutures are placed at the level of the midurethra and a second pair at the vesical neck.

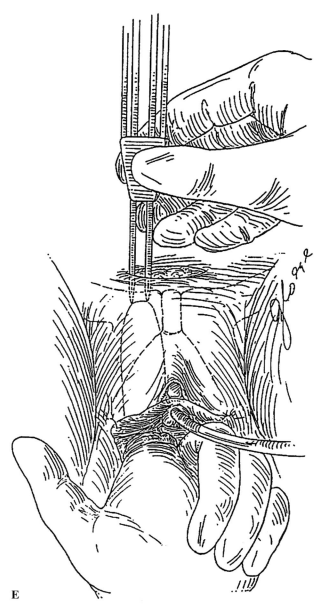

E

E: A small suprapubic incision is made and an index finger is advanced into the vaginal wound retracting the bladder and urethra medially. The undersurface of the rectus fascia is indented with the tip of the finger and a needle carrier is advanced into the vaginal wound. The long ends of the suture are threaded through the needle and pulled into the abdominal wound.

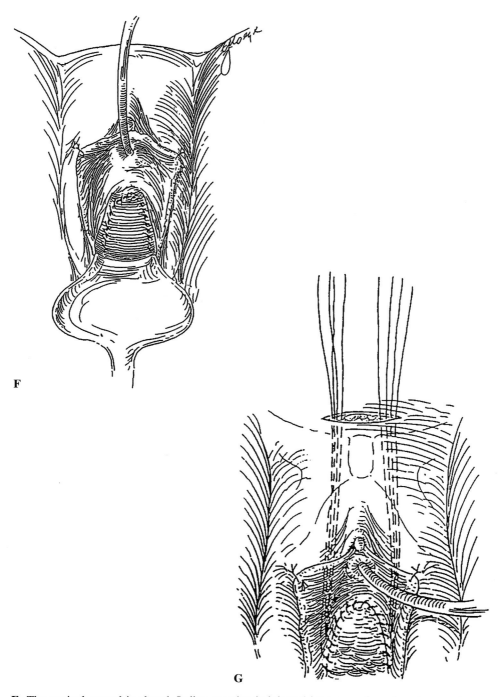

F: The vaginal wound is closed. Indigo carmine is injected intravenously and cystoscopy is performed to be sure there has been no injury to the bladder, urethra, or ureters. Efflux of blue urine from each ureter assures their patency. G: The long ends of the sutures are tied above the fascia in the midline with no added tension. (From Walsh et al., ref. 45, with permission.)

vation or strengthening of the periurethral tissues is accomplished and there may be no improvement in incontinence. Moreover, the tissue pass is blind, there is no way of determining the exact needle placement, and it is necessary to perform cystoscopy to ensure that there has not been inadvertent entry into the bladder or urethra.

Leach has modified the Raz[39] procedure further by securing the ends of the suture to the pubic bone instead of tying them together over the rectus fascia. He believes that this maneuver reduces the likelihood of troublesome suprapubic pain which, in his experience, had been a complication of concern.

RETROPUBIC URETHROPEXY

Retropubic urethropexy was first described in the adult in 1949 by Marshall et al.[40] Their first patient, interestingly, was a man who had developed stress incontinence after undergoing abdominal perineal resection of the rectum. All of the retropubic urethropexies have the common goal of identifying strong periurethral tissues near the vesical neck and suturing them to a strong supporting structure or tissue attached to the pubis. Ideally, the sutures transverse the strong periurethral tissue by taking a nearly full thickness bite of vaginal wall excluding the vaginal epithelium. This bite should include the levator complex with its attendant fascia. In the Marshall-Marchetti-Krantz operation (Fig. 5.4) this tissue is fixed to the undersurface of the pubis. In the Burch repair[41] (Fig. 5.5) it is fixed to

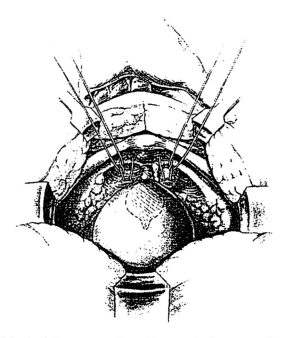

Fig. 5.4. Marshall-Marchetti-Krantz procedure. Exposure is the same as in the Burch procedure. Paired sutures are placed on either side of the vesical neck and proximal urethra and tied to the periosteum and cartilage of the symphysis pubis. (From Walthers and Karram, ref. 40a, with permission.)

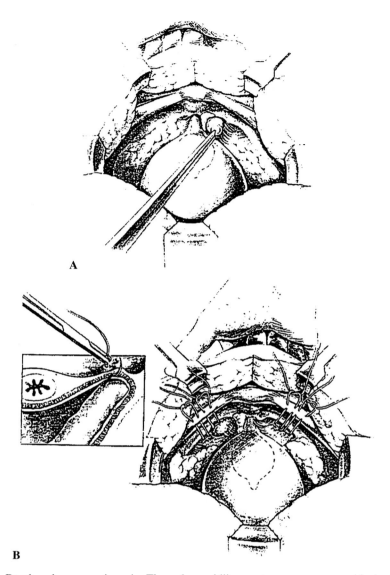

Fig. 5.5. Burch culposuspension. **A:** Through a midline or transverse suprapubic incision, the retropubic space is entered and the peritoneum reflected superiorly. The glistening white surface of the endopelvic fascia is identified with a combination of blunt and sharp dissection. This maneuver is facilitated by indenting the vaginal wall lateral to the vesical neck with an index finger in the vagina. **B:** Several full-thickness bites of the vaginal wall, excluding the epithelium are taken adjacent to the vesical neck and passed through Cooper's ligament on either side. The sutures are all passed, then tied while the index finger elevates the vagina. (From Walthers and Karram, ref. 40a, with permission.)

Cooper's ligament, and in the paravaginal repair of Richardson,[42] it is sutured to the arcus tendineus (Fig. 5.6). Some authors recommend that only nonabsorbable sutures be used in these repairs, such as silk or mersilene; others advocate absorbable "chromic catgut" or long lasting absorbable sutures such as polyglycolic (Dexon) or polydioxanone (PDS).

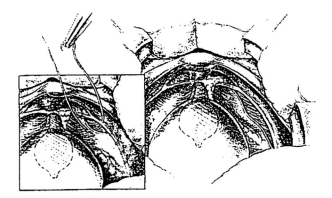

Fig. 5.6. Richardson paravaginal repair. Through a retropubic incision, the lateral edge of the defect in the endopelvic fascia is sutured to the arcus tendineus fasciae pelvis. (From Walthers and Karram, ref. 40a, with permission.)

Recently there has been a resurgence of interest in the Burch procedure performed through a laparascope, avoiding an abdominal incision. However, the advantages of reduced hospital stay, decreased use of narcotics, and early return to work must be weighed against the unknown results.

PUBOVAGINAL SLING

Pubovaginal sling has gained recent popularity as the treatment of choice for intrinsic sphincter deficiency, but we recommend it with equal enthusiasm for patients with ure-thral hypermobility. We prefer to harvest the sling from the rectus abdominus fas-cia[4,6,9,11,14,43,44] due to the ease of accessibility at the time of surgery, but others have recommended fascia lata[4,10,15,16] or synthetics including mersilene, dacron, and Mar-lex.[7,8,12,13,17,18] No matter what technique is used it is important to position the sling around the vesical neck with no tension at all. Tension on the sling results in urinary obstruction and/or detrusor instability. Our technique for pubovaginal sling is depicted in Fig. 5.7.

POSTOPERATIVE CARE

The general principles of postoperative care are the same for all of the procedures described above. An indwelling cathether is left in place until a voiding trial commences, usually in the first 1–5 days. When concomitant prolapse surgery is done, it usually takes a bit longer before the patient is voiding well. Either a urethral (Foley) catheter or supra-pubic tube may be used. We prefer the latter because it is much easier to manage the void-ing trial by having the patient open and close the suprapubic catheter than by having the patient or staff repeatedly catheterize in the early postoperative period. Some surgeons routinely start the patient on intermittent catheterization soon after surgery, but we prefer to wait until the vaginal incisions are healing well. If the patient voids satisfactorily and there is not excessive residual urine, the catheter is removed. If not, the tube is left in place and another voiding trial is undertaken in 2 to 4 weeks.

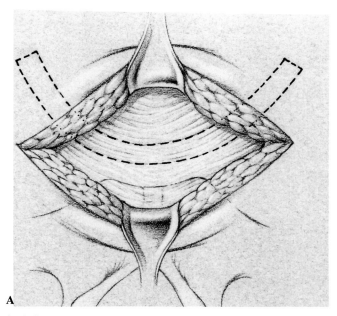

Fig. 5.7. Pubovaginal (fascial) sling. **A:** Pfannenstiel skin incision is made and carried down to the rectus fascia. The surface of the rectus fascia is dissected free of subcutaneous tissue and a suitable site is selected for excision of the fascial strip which will be used as a free graft for creation of the sling. Two parallel horizontal incisions, 2 –3 cm apart, are made near the midline in the rectus fascia. The incisions are extended superiorly and laterally for the entire width of the wound, following the direction of the fascial fibers. This usually results in a sling of about 18 cm in length, but it is not necessary for the sling to be long enough to reach the rectus fascia on either side.

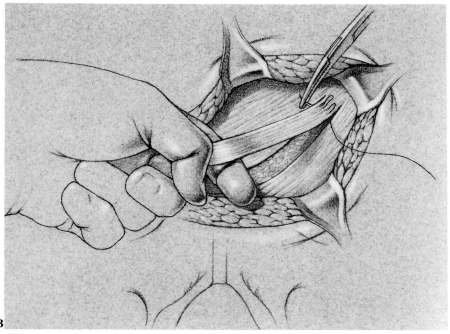

B: Before excising the strip, each end of the fascia is secured with a long 2-0 monofilament nonabsorbable suture using a running horizontal mattress which is placed at right angles to the direction of the fascial fibers.

101

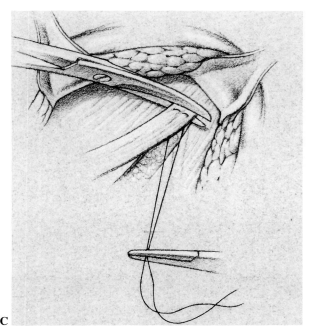

C: Each end of the fascial strip is transected approximately 1 cm lateral to the sutures and placed in a basin of saline.

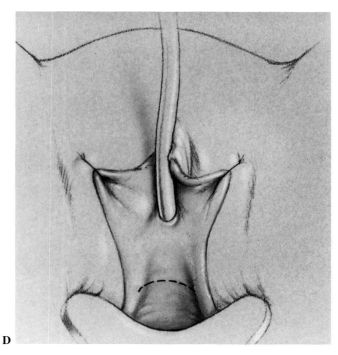

D: A 4-cm, slightly curved, horizontal incision is made over the vesical neck and a small vaginal flap, about 2 cm wide, is elevated.

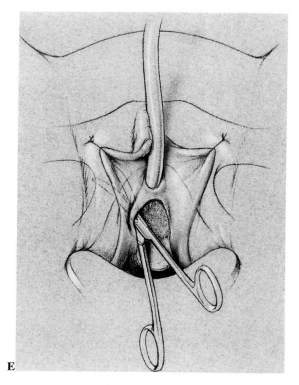

E

E: The lateral edges of the vaginal wound are grasped with Allis clamps and retracted laterally. The dissection continues just beneath the vaginal epithelium with a Metzenbaum scissors pointed in the direction of the patient's ipsilateral shoulder until the periosteum of the pubis or ischium is palpated with the tip of the scissors. During this part of the dissection, it is important to stay as far laterally as possible. This is best accomplished by dissecting with the concavity of the scissor pointing laterally and by exerting constant lateral pressure with the tips of the scissor against the undersurface of the vaginal epithelium.

During this part of the dissection, the proper plane is confirmed by palpation with an index finger. The tip of the finger, opposite the nail, palpates the periosteium. With the back edge of the fingertip the bladder and urethra are mobilized medially as the finger advances and perforates the fascia. This completely mobilizes the vesical neck and proximal urethra releasing these structures from their vaginal attachments. In some instances this dissection must be performed sharply with Metzenbaum scissors. The surgeon's right index finger is reinserted in the vaginal wound retracting the vesical neck and bladder medially. The tip of the finger indents the undersurface of the rectus and is palpated by the index finger of the left hand in the abdominal wound.

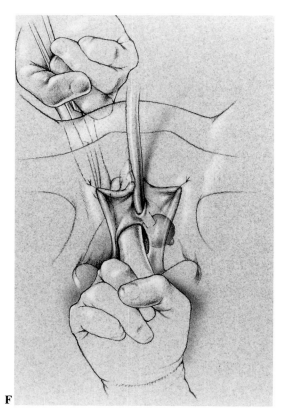

F: A long sharp curved clamp (DeBakey) is inserted into the incision and directed to the undersurface of the pubis. The tip of the clamp is pressed against the periosteum and directed toward the index finger which is retracting the vesical neck and bladder medially. The clamp is guided into the vaginal wound.

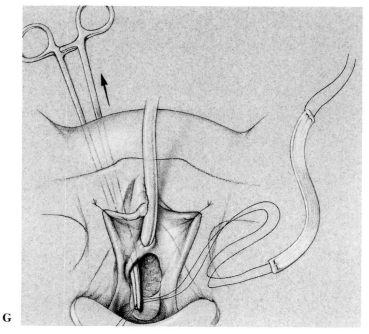

G: When the tip of the clamp is visible, one end of the long suture, which is attached to the fascial graft, is grasped and pulled into the abdominal wound. The procedure is repeated on the other side. Indigo carmine is given intravenously and cystoscopy performed. The vaginal incision is closed.

104

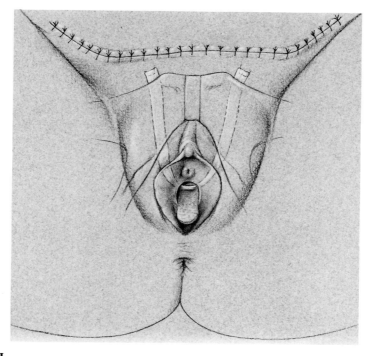

H

H: The fascial sling is now positioned from the abdominal wall on one side around the undersurface of the vesical neck and back to the abdominal wall on the other side. A small incision is made in the inferior leaf of the rectus fascia on either side and the long sutures attached to either end of the sling are pulled through. The rectus fascia is closed with a running 2:0 absorbable monfilament suture. The two long sutures are tied together in the midline over the rectus fascia without any tension at all. (From Blaivas and Jacobs, ref 6, with permission.)

RESULTS

With the exception of the Kelly plication, all of the procedures discussed above have a 1-year cure rate ranging from 80 to 95%. Long-term data is very sparse in the literature; only the Burch procedure and pubovaginal sling have any meaningful studies and these show 5-year cure rates of over 80%.[13,30] A few reports on long-term results of the transvaginal urethropexies show disappointing cure rates of about 50%.[32,34]

Complications

There is a paucity of reports in the literature on complications of the aforementioned operations. What follows is a discussion based on what little there is in the literature and the authors' not entirely unbiased opinions. The most devastating complications (aside from death which occurs in about 0.02%) are vesicovaginal and urethrovaginal fistula and ureteral injury which are quite rare, occurring in well under 1% of patients. Most of these occur (1) when nonabsorbable, braided sutures such as silk inadvertently traverse the bladder, urethra, or ureter during Marshall-Marchetti-Krantz or Burch procedures, (2) when nonabsorbable synthetic mesh is used as a bolster for needle urethropexies, (3) when nonabsorbable synthetic mesh is used for a synthetic pubovaginal sling, or (4) when the sutures from a Kelly plication are tied too tightly around a Foley catheter which is left in the urethra too long.

The next most troublesome complications are urinary retention and symptomatic detrusor instability. Data on the likelihood of these occurring are sparse, but a recent review of the literature suggests that about 3% of patients after urethropexy operations and 7% after pubovaginal sling develop permanent urinary retention requiring either intermittent self-catheterization or urethrolysis. Refractory symptoms of detrusor instability occur in about 10% of patients regardless of the type of operation. Both of these complications are largely preventable as they occur when the sutures used for the repair are tied too tightly.

REFERENCES

1. Parnell JP, Marshall VF, Vaughan ED: Primary management of urinary stress incontinence by the Marshall-Marchetti-Krantz vesicourethropexy. *J Urol* 127:679, 1982.

2. Varner RE, Sparks JM: Surgery for stress urinary incontinence. *Surg Clin North Am* 71:1111–1134, 1991.

3. Kirby RS, Whiteway JE: Assessment of the results of Stamey bladder neck suspension. *Br J Urol* 63:21–23, 1989.

4. Awad SA, Flood HD, Acker KL: The significance of prior anti-incontinence surgery in women who present with urinary incontinence. *J Urol* 140:514, 1988.

5. Beck RP, McCormick S, Nordstrom L: The fascia lata sling procedure for treating recurrent genuine stress incontinence of urine. *Obstet Gynecol* 72:699, 1988.

6. Blaivas JG, Jacobs BZ: Pubovaginal fascial sling for the treatment of complicated stress urinary incontinence. *J Urol* 145:1214, 1991.

7. Bryans FE: Marlex gauze hammock sling operation with Cooper's ligament attachment in the management of recurrent urinary stress incontinence. *Am J Obstet Gynecol* 133:292, 1979.

8. Fianu S, Soderberg G: Absorbable polyglactin mesh for retropubic sling operations in female stress urinary incontinence. *Gynecol Obstet Invest* 16:45, 1983.

9. Hohenfellner T, Petri E. In Stanton SL, Tanagho EA (eds): *Surgery of Female Incontinence.* Berlin, Springer-Verlag, 1980.

10. Low JA: Management of severe anatomic deficiencies of urethral sphincter function by a combined procedure with a fascia lata sling. *Am J Obstet Gynecol* 105:149, 1969.

11. McGuire EJ, Lytton B: Pubovaginal sling procedures for stress incontinence. *J Urol* 119:82, 1978.

12. Moir JC: The gauze-hammock operation (a modified Aldride sling procedure) *J Obstet Gynaecol Br Commonwealth* 75:1, 1968.

13. Morgan JE, Farrow GA, Stewart FE: The Marlex sling operation for the treatment of recurrent stress urinary incontinence: a 16-year review. *Am J Obstet Gynecol* 151:224, 1985.

14. Narik B, Palmrich A: A simplified sling operation suitable for routine use. *Am J Obstet Gynecol* 84:400–405, 1962.

15. Parker RT, Adison WA, Wilson CJ: Fascia lata urethrovesical suspension for recurrent stress urinary incontinence. *Am J Obstet Gynecol* 135:843, 1979.

16. Ridley JH: The Goebel-Stoeckel sling operation. In Mattingly RF, Thompson JD (eds): *Telinde's Operative Gynecology.* Philadelphia, Lippincott, 1985, pp 623–636.

17. Stanton SL, Brindley GS, Holmes DM: Silastic sling for urethral sphincter incompetence in women. *Br J Obstet Gynaecol* 92:747, 1985.

18. Williams TJ, Telinde RW: The sling operation for urinary incontinence using mersilene ribbon. *Obstet Gynecol* 19:241, 1962.

19. Appell RA: Techniques and results in the implantation of the artificial urinary sphincter in women with type III stress urinary incontinence by a vaginal approach. *Neurol Urodyn* 7:613, 1988.

20. Scott FB: The use of the artificial sphincter in the treatment of urinary incontinence in the female patient. *Urol Clin North Am* 12:305, 1985.

21. Santarosa RP, Blaivas JG: Periurethral injection of autologous fat for treatment of sphincteric incontinence. *J Urol* 151:607, 1994.

22. Herschorn S, Radomski SB, Steele DJ: Early experience with intraurethral collagen injections for urinary incontinence. *J Urol* 148:1797, 1992.

23. McGuire EJ, Appell RA: Transurethral collagen injection for urinary incontinence. *Urology* 43:413–415, 1994.

24. Buckley JF, Scott R, Lingham V, et al: Injectable silicone microparticles: a new treatment for female stress incontinence. *J Urol* 147:280A, 1992.

25. Blaivas JG, Olsson CA: Stress incontinence: classification and surgical approach. *J Urol* 139:727, 1988.

26. Kelly HA, Dumm WM: Urinary incontinence in women, without manifest injury to the bladder. *Surg Gynecol Obstet* 18:444–450, 1914.

26a. Nichols DH, Randall CL: *Vaginal Surgery*, ed 3, Baltimore, Williams & Wilkins, 1989.

27. Wall LL, Norton PA, DeLancey JOL: *Practical Urogynecology*. Baltimore, Williams & Wilkins, 1993, pp 153–190.

28. Stanton SI, Cardozo LD: A comparison of vaginal and suprapubic surgery in the correction of incontinence due to urethral sphincter incompetence. *Br J Urol* 59:497, 1979.

29. Park GS, Miller EJ Jr: Surgical treatment of stress urinary incontinence: a comparison of the Kelly plication, Marshall-Marchetti-Krantz, and Pereyra operations. *Obstet Gynecol* 71:575, 1988.

30. van Geelen JM, Theeuwes AG, Eskes TK, et al: The clinical and urodynamic effects of anterior vaginal repair and Burch colposuspension. *Am J Obstet Gynecol* 159:137, 1988.

31. Thunedborg P, Fischer-Rasmussen W, Jensen SB: Stress urinary incontinence and posterior bladder suspension defects. Results of vaginal repair versus Burch colposuspension. *Acta Obstet Gynecol Scand* 69:55, 1990.

32. Bergman A, Ballard CA, Koonings PP: Comparison of three different surgical procedures for genuine stress incontinence: prospective randomized study. *Am J Obstet Gynecol* 160:1102, 1989.

33. Siegel AL, Raz S: Surgical treatment of anatomical stress incontinence. *Neurol Urodyn* 7:569–583, 1988.

34. Kelly MJ, Knielsen K, Bruskewitz R, et al: Symptom analysis of patients undergoing modified Pereyra bladder neck suspension for stress urinary incontinence. *Urology* 37:213–219, 1991.

35. Pereyra AJ: A simplified surgical procedure for the correction of stress incontinence in women. *West Surg Obstet Gynecol* 67:223, 1959.

36. Stamey TA: Endoscopic suspension of the vesical neck for urinary incontinence in females: a report on 203 consecutive patients. *Ann Surg* 192:465, 1980.

37. Cobb OE, Radge H: Simplified correction of female stress incontinence. *J Urol* 120:418, 1978.

38. Gittes RF, Loughlin KR: No-incision pubovaginal suspension for stress incontinence. *J Urol* 138:568, 1987.

39. Raz S: Modified bladder neck suspension for female stress incontinence. *Urology* 17:82, 1981.

40. Marshall VF, Marchetti AA, Krantz KE: The correction of stress incontinence by simple vesicourethral suspension. *Surg Gynecol Obstet* 88:509, 1949.

40a. Walthers MD, Genuine Stress Incontinence: Retropubic Surgical Procedures. In: Walthers MD, Karram MM. *Clinical Urogynecology*, St. Louis, Mosby–Year Book, Inc., 1993.

41. Burch JC: Urethrovaginal fixation to Cooper's ligament for correction of stress incontinence, cystocele, and prolapse. *Am J Obstet Gynecol* 81:281, 1961.

42. Richardson AC, Edmonds PB, Williams NL: Treatment of stress urinary incontinence due to paravaginal fascial defect. *Obstet Gynecol* 57:357, 1981.

43. Blaivas JG, Salinas J: Type III stress urinary incontinence: importance of proper diagnosis and treatment. *Surg Forum* 35:473, 1984.

44. McGuire EJ, Lytton B: Pubovaginal sling procedures for stress incontinence. *J Urol* 145:1214, 1991.

45. Walsh PC, Gittes RF, Perlmutter AD, et al: *Campbell's Urology,* ed 6. Philadelphia, WB Saunders, 1992.

6

Surgery for Sphincteric Incontinence in Males

François Haab
Gary E. Leach

Urinary continence in males is dependent upon two functional areas: (1) the proximal urethral sphincteric mechanism centered at the bladder neck and including the prostate gland and the prostatic urethra to the verumontanum, (2) the distal urethral sphincter extending from the verumontanum to the bulbar urethra.[1] The distal urethral sphincter has three principal components: the intrinsic smooth muscle layer, the intrinsic rhabdosphincter capable of maintaining a baseline tone over prolonged period, and the extrinsic skeletal muscle layer. This extrinsic skeletal muscle is composed of fast-twich fibers which supplement the activity of the rhabdosphincter under stress conditions.[1] The proximal urethral sphincter is mainly innervated by adrenergic fibers.[2] The innervation of the striated external urethral sphincter is still debated but probably combines somatic nerves via the pudendal nerve and autonomic nerves via the pelvic plexus.[3] Either the proximal or the distal urethral sphincteric mechanisms must be functionally intact to maintain continence.

The most common cause of male stress urinary incontinence (SUI) is sphincteric damage during prostatectomy. Postprostatectomy incontinence occurs in less than 1% of surgery for benign prostatic hyperplasia treatment and this complication ranges from 2% to 87% of men following radical prostatectomy.[4–6] In a review on 757 Medicare patients who had undergone radical prostatectomy, 47% of survey respondents had urinary leakage every day, and 32% required protection or a penile clamp. Six percent of survey respondents required another surgical procedure to correct their urinary incontinence.[7] Over half of the men who reported wearing pads after radical prostatectomy considered their incontinence to be a "medium" or "big" problem with a negative effect on quality of life.[8,9]

Sphincteric incompetence following prostatectomy for benign disease can be iatrogenic (i.e., direct damage to the distal urethral sphincter) or can result from preexisting denervation of the distal urethral sphincter. Such denervation should be suspected in men after radical pelvic surgery (i.e., abdominal perineal resection of the rectum), pelvic trauma, pelvic radiation, or urethroplasty.[10,11] Based on our experience, urinary incontinence after radical prostatectomy is caused by bladder dysfunction, sphincteric insufficiency, or both.[12–16] Therefore it is extremely important that any treatment for postprostatectomy incontinence be directed by appropriate urodynamic studies.

The purpose of this chapter is to present and discuss the most commonly used surgical techniques to correct sphincteric incontinence in men.

ARTIFICIAL URINARY SPHINCTER

The artificial urinary sphincter (AUS) is the most commonly used surgical procedure to correct urinary incontinence related to sphincteric dysfunction in men. The results of AUS placement are directly related to proper patient selection.

Patient Selection

The ideal candidate for AUS placement has normal detrusor function and compliance, with incontinence secondary to sphincteric incompetence alone. The criteria for AUS insertion are strict and are summarized in Table 6.1.

In our experience, the presence of incontinence after prostatectomy is not synonymous with stress incontinence caused by sphincteric damage.[13] We recently reviewed the urodynamic records of 215 men with postprostatectomy incontinence. In the cancer group (n = 159), 40% of the patients had stress incontinence alone, whereas 56% had a major component of high-pressure bladder dysfunction contributing to their urinary incontinence. The urodynamic findings were similar in the benign group.[17] These findings underscore the importance of urodynamic evaluation prior to AUS placement, with special attention to bladder function. A treatment algorithm, based on urodynamic findings is depicted in Fig. 6.1. When detrusor instability and/or poor bladder wall compliance is associated with SUI, an initial attempt is made to "normalize" the intravesical pressure with anticholinergic therapy. When significant SUI persists while on anticholinergic therapy, the urodynamic evaluation should be repeated to confirm low bladder pressures and significant SUI before AUS insertion. When anticholinergic treatment is unsuccessful in controlling high bladder pressures, augmentation cystoplasty with a detubularized intestinal segment should be considered.[12,17] The risks of infection, mechanical failure, reoperation, persistent or recurrent stress incontinence, and removal of the device should be clearly discussed as part of preoperative informed consent.

TABLE 6.1. Criteria of Eligibility for Artificial Urinary Sphincter Placement

Significant urinary incontinence (>2 pads/day)
Duration of incontinence of at least 12 months
No response to pharmacologic therapy
Sterile urine
Unobstructed flow
Stable bladder
Patient motivated
Manual dexterity

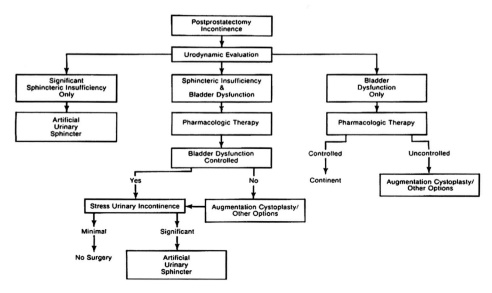

Fig. 6.1. Suggested algorithm for the management of postprostatectomy incontinence.

Technical Aspects

Preoperative Preparation

Patients scheduled for AUS placement are admitted to the hospital the morning of the surgical procedure. We routinely instruct patients to perform an antiseptic scrub of the lower abdomen, genitals, and perineum the evening before and the morning of the surgery. Broad-spectrum intravenous antibiotics are administered perioperatively and for 24 h postoperatively, and then orally for at least 4 days after surgery. The patient is shaved in the operative room to prevent bacterial colonization of skin abrasions. Draping is completed with isolation of the rectum from the operative field.

Operative Procedure

The patient is placed in the modified lithotomy position: one leg is lowered to gain access to the lower abdomen on the side of reservoir placement. A 16-Fr silicone Foley catheter is inserted. A midline perineal incision is used to expose the bulbar urethra, and the Scott ring retractor is used to maintain good exposure. During dissection, palpation of the catheter helps to identify the urethra. After separation of the bulbocavernosous muscle, the bulbar urethra is mobilized circumferentially for a distance of 2 cm. Care must be taken to avoid entering the urethra anteriorly, especially in patients with a history of pelvic radiation. Should the urethra be injured, the defect may be closed with a 4-0 adsorbable suture and the cuff may be placed in another more distal area. The properly sized cuff, which for the bulbar urethra is almost always 4.5 cm, is passed around the urethra.

An abdominal transverse incision is made just above the inguinal ligament. The external oblique fascia is exposed and incised. The reservoir is placed in a preperitoneal pocket created beneath the abdominal muscles with the tubing exiting through the incision site.

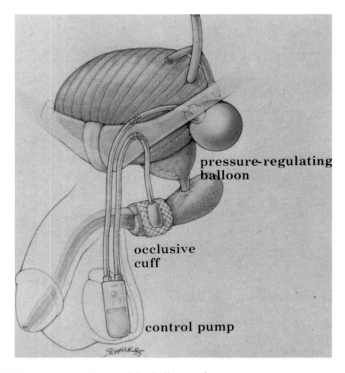

Fig. 6.2. AMS 800 device placed around the bulbar urethra.

The fascia is closed with preplaced sutures to avoid injury to the reservoir. The reservoir is filled with the appropriate volume (23 cc) of iso-osmotic contrast material. We routinely use the 51–60 cm pressure reservoir to minimize the risk of urethral atrophy. The pump is placed in a lateral subdartos pouch created in the dependent scrotum. Appropriate tubing connections are made and the sphincter function is checked by performing intraoperative sphincterometry. Fig. 6.2 depicts the positioning of the prosthesis.

   We routinely use intraoperative perfusion sphincterometry to document appropriate function of the device and also to identify any unrecognized urethral injury.[18] Perfusion sphincterometry is performed by placing an 8-Fr pediatric Foley catheter in the meatus and inflating the balloon in the fossa navicularis to occlude the urethra. Indigo carmine stained fluid is used to perfuse the urethra. The bag of stained saline is raised until the fluid level at the top of the bag is 51 cm above the level of the cuff. Once the urethral segment between the closed cuff and occluded meatus is filled with fluid, the infusion should stop. The pump is then squeezed to open the cuff and allow infusion to resume. The time until the cuff reinflates and infusion again stops is noted. The cuff reinflation time should be between 3 to 5 min. The height of the bag is then slowly raised until the fluid begins to drop. The height at which fluid infusion resumes represents the cuff closure pressure. This pressure should correlate with the pressure range of the balloon (51–60 cm water). To exclude the possibility of urethral injury, a white gauze is placed in the perineal incision. Any evidence of a blue stain on the white gauze may indicate the presence of urethral injury.

After perfusion sphincterometry is completed, the incisions are closed, the device is deactivated, and a condom catheter is placed. A radiograph is performed in the recovery room to confirm contrast in the AUS and a normal appearance for all components.

Bladder Neck Cuff Placement

The bladder neck approach is preferred in young patients, patients with SUI on a neurogenic basis, or when the bulbar urethra is severely scarred. the bladder neck is exposed through a subumbilical midline incision. The cuff is positioned between the seminal vesicles and bladder neck with the bladder open to improve exposure.[19] The bladder neck is circumferentially measured and an appropriately sized cuff is placed. A 71- to 80-cm water pressure reservoir is generally used.

Postoperative Care

As soon as possible, the patient is taught to pull down the pump to maintain it in the most dependent scrotal position. Patients wear diapers or condom drainage devices during the period of deactivation. When scrotal pain and swelling are resolved, the device is activated (usually 4 to 8 weeks after the operation).

Should postoperative urinary retention occur, clean intermittent catheterization with a 12- or 14-Fr catheter is performed.

Results

Successful treatment of urinary incontinence can be achieved in 60% to 80% of the patients with AUS placement (Table 6.2).[20–23] We recently reviewed our treatment outcome in 135 men with postprostatectomy incontinence. Based on the urodynamic evaluation, an AUS was inserted in 56 men with SUI. Seventeen of these 56 patients were first treated with anticholinergic therapy because of bladder dysfunction with SUI. Evaluation of the severity of incontinence before and after AUS placement was based upon a numerical pad scoring system (No protection required = 0, < 2 pads per day = 1, 2–4 pads per day = 2, and > 4 pads per day = 3). Overall treatment results for both the cancer group and the benign group demonstrated a significant decrease in the pad score for those who underwent AUS placement and those who had their high-pressure bladder dysfunction controlled pharmacologically prior to AUS insertion (Fig. 6.3). Gundian et al. recently reported 87% of men were satisfied after AUS insertion to correct postprostatectomy incontinence.[24] In our experience, men with very significant postprostatectomy incontinence are most satisfied with AUS placement.

TABLE 6.2. Continence Rate after Artificial Urinary Sphincter Placement

	Perez[20] (n = 75)	Leo[21] (n = 136)	Light[22] (n = 88)	Montague[23] (n = 156)
Follow-up (months)	44 (5–116)	28	35 (4–82)	41 (6–94)
No pad	78%	81%	81%	81%
<2 pad/day	9%	11%	13%	12%
>2 pad/day	13%	8%	6%	5%
Total incontinent	0%	0%	0%	2%

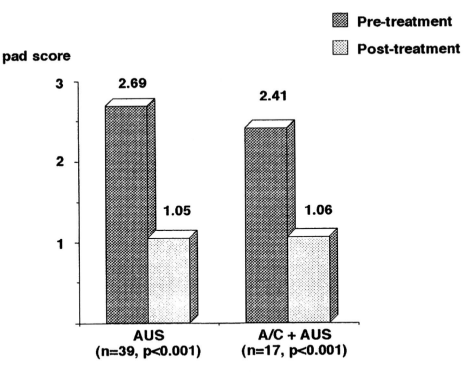

Fig. 6.3. Postprostatectomy incontinence: treatment results. AUS = artificial urinary sphincter; A/C = anticholinergic).

The continence rate was found to be lower in neurogenic patients because of bladder dysfunction as well as in the irradiated patients due to urethral erosion.[25]

Complications

With appropriate patient selection, perioperative care, and surgical technique, AUS placement can be accomplished with minimal morbidity.

Mechanical Failure

The revision rate related to mechanical failure ranges between 4% and 30%, however the rate of mechanical failure has decreased considerably since three component modifications have been made: kink resistant tubing, "suture-less" tubing connectors, and a silicone surface treated cuff to prevent cuff leakage (Table 6.3).[20–23] The latest model AMS 800 device has been estimated to have a reliability rate of 95% over a 36-month period, with most failures related to fluid leak from the cuff.[26]

Device Removal (Infection, Erosion)

Cuff erosion and/or infection has been reported in 8% to 13% of adults undergoing implantation of AMS 800. The mean explanation rate is 8%, which is mainly related to erosion and infection (Table 6.4).[20–23] Patients with a history of prior urethral surgery or radiation

TABLE 6.3. AUS Placement: Cause of Reoperation for Mechanical Failure

	Perez[20] (n = 75)	Leo[21] (n = 136)	Light[22] (n = 88)	Montague[23] (n = 156)
Follow-up (months)	44 (5–116)	28	35 (4–82)	41 (6–94)
Tube kinking	8%	4%	0%	3%
Cuff leak	17%	2.7%	1.3%	1.8%
Reservoir leak	4%	0.7%	0%	1.2%
Connector leak	0%	3.5%	0%	1.2%
Pump failure	4%	1.4%	2.3%	1.2%

therapy are at increased risk for cuff erosion.[20,24,25] In our experience, cuff erosion is frequently caused by urethral catheterization through a closed cuff. Symptoms of cuff erosion may include pain and swelling in the perineum or scrotum, recurrent urinary incontinence, urinary tract infection, or bloody urethral discharge. The diagnosis of cuff erosion is confirmed with urethrography and urethroscopy. Treatment requires cuff removal, and a silicone catheter is inserted for 3 weeks. When there is no gross evidence of infection, the remaining components of the device may be left in situ with stainless steel plug occlusion of the tubing and prolonged postoperative antibiotics.[27] After waiting 3 to 6 months, the author will consider a new cuff placement at a different urethral site. However, in our experience, erosion of the cuff into the urethra is in most cases associated with a chronically infected device, necessitating removal of the entire AUS. Hopefully, reimplantation after adequate treatment of the infection is successful in the majority of patients.

Incontinence

Persistent or transient urinary incontinence has been described in 20% to 30% of the patients after AUS placement.[20–23] This incontinence may be caused by bladder dysfunction, malfunction of the device, cuff erosion, or local urethral atrophy underneath the cuff.

We follow a simple protocol, based on physical examination, cystometry, radiograph evaluation, cystoscopy, and retrograde perfusion sphincterometry (Fig. 6.4).[28] In the office, we first pump the device. Inability to compress the pump may be caused by a tubing kink, obstructed system, or fluid loss. The cuff assembly should be examined with an inflate/deflate radiograph to be sure that the device has not been accidentally deactivated and that there is no fluid loss. Slight loss of fluid can be associated with an abnormal "pear shaped" balloon. Recently, ultrasound examination was proposed as a more sensitive test than standard radiographs to assess the volume of fluid in the reservoir.[29] When the radi-

TABLE 6.4. AUS: Causes for Removal of the Device (NA: not available)

	Perez[20] (n = 75)	Leo[21] (n = 136)	Light[22] (n = 88)	Montague[23] (n = 156)
Follow-up (months)	44 (5–116)	28	35 (4–82)	41 (6–94)
Erosion	5.4%	2%	NA	6%
Infection	0%	0%	7%	1.2%
Other	2.6%	2%	0%	0.6%

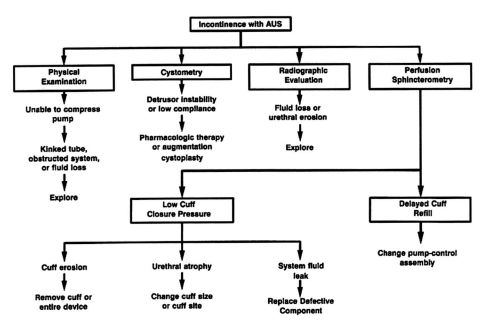

Fig. 6.4. Algorithm for evaluation of incontinence after artificial urinary sphincter (AUS) placement.

ographic appearance of the device is normal, cystourethroscopy and a retrograde urethrogram are performed to exclude urethral erosion of the cuff. When there is no evidence of mechanical failure or cuff erosion, a cystometrogram is performed to confirm normal bladder pressures. Bladder dysfunction can either be present before AUS placement or can develop after insertion of the device.[28,30] Therefore, an in-depth urodynamic evaluation to evaluate bladder function in patients incontinent after AUS placement is of utmost importance. Finally we perform a retrograde perfusion sphincterometry (utilizing the same technique as employed intraoperatively) to measure the cuff closure pressure, to confirm cuff deflation, and to define the time required for cuff reinflation.[28] A low closure pressure may be caused by urethral atrophy, cuff erosion, or a fluid leak. A small urethral erosion may be diagnosed only with intraoperative perfusion sphincterometry with indigo carmine stained fluid after the cuff is exposed.[28]

    Management of urethral atrophy at the cuff site is challenging. The reported incidence of this complication is 7% to 15% but may be less since the introduction of the narrow back cuff in 1987.[21] In our practice, we have attempted to delay or prevent urethral atrophy by routine use of the low-pressure 51–60 cm water-pressure-regulating reservoir. Several treatments have been proposed to address urethral atrophy: move the cuff more distally to a normal segment of the urethra, to increase the pressure of the reservoir, to decrease the cuff size at the original cuff site, or to insert a second cuff.[31–33] In our practice we prefer to move the cuff more distally since we are concerned that increasing the pressure exerted on the already thin urethra may increase the risk of cuff erosion after placement of a higher pressure balloon. When there is no erosion or infection, incontinence after AUS placement can be managed successfully in 80% to 90% of the patients.[30]

BULKING AGENTS

Transurethral injection of various materials has been used to increase urethral resistance and correct stress urinary incontinence in males.

Materials Used

Teflon paste or polytetrafluoroethylene (Polytef) consists of 4- to 1-μm particles, and has been used for transurethral injections over the past 20 years.[34] However, Teflon has not achieved universal acceptance because of its high cost, difficulty with injection, documented migration, and local complications.[35] Polytef has never been approved by the U.S. Food and Drug Administration (FDA) for transurethral injections to treat urinary incontinence.

Recently the FDA has approved glutaraldehyde crosslinked, highly purified, bovine dermal collagene (GAX-collagen) for periurethral injections. Although purified bovine collagen appears to have improved compatibility over the earlier material, allergic reactions occurs in 1.4% to 3% of the patients.[36] Moreover, periurethral collagen injections are expensive. Compared to the AUS, collagen is a more expensive method to treat urinary incontinence in males.[37]

Transurethral autologous fat injection was first introduced in 1989 by Santiago de Garibay as an inexpensive, biocompatible, and readily available periurethral bulking agent.[38] Fat is harvested from the lower abdominal wall using a liposuction technique.[39] Thirty milliliters of fat are obtained and washed with normal saline. The procedure is performed under local anesthesia.

Technique of Periurethral Injection

Preoperative Preparation

Patients should be taught self-catheterization preoperatively to manage any transient postoperative urinary retention. Sterility of the urine should be ensured. Patients should also be fully informed about the potential complications of the procedure, including immediate failure, recurrent urinary incontinence necessitating repeated injections, transient urinary retention, and, in case of fat harvesting, donor site pain, bruising, and rarely hematoma or infection. All patients who are candidates for GAX-collagen should be skin-tested 1 month before treatment.

Transurethral Injection Technique

Bulking agents should be injected in the narrow urethral segment above the external sphincter and not directly into the external sphincter.[40]

The patient is placed in a semilithotomy position. Local anesthesia is performed with 2% lidocaine jelly transurethrally and 5 to 10 ml of 1% plain lidocaine injected through the perineum. Cystourethroscopy is performed with a 21-Fr sheath and 0 degree lens, allowing injection under direct visual control. The injection needle is placed transurethrally via a special scope and the material is injected until the urethral mucosa nearly coapts in the midline. Several injection sites are usually required.

Recently, a transperineal approach under transrectal ultrasound guidance was described with a cure rate similar to those of previous reports.[41]

Results

Treatment of postprostatectomy sphincteric incontinence with periurethral injections has been disappointing regardless of the substance injected. Using periurethral polytetrafluoroethylene injections in 13 men with postprostatectomy incontinence, Kabalin recently reported that only 23% of the patients experienced significant improvement of continence status, 77% experienced no improvement in continence, and no men were completely dry at 1-year follow-up.[42] Conversely Politano reported an improvement in 80% of men with postprostatectomy incontinence.[43] However the evaluation criteria and length of follow-up were not clearly defined.

Periurethral collagen injections for postprostatectomy incontinence have a cure/improvement rate ranging between 40% and 60% of the patients at 1-year follow-up, with few men being totally dry.[37,40,41,44,45] Most patients need more than two injections with a cumulative mean volume injected of 25 cc (Table 6.5). Liu et al. found no correlation between outcome after collagen injection and age, Vasalva leak point pressure, initial grade of incontinence, history of transient dryness, or urinary retention after the first session.[44] Conversely, McGuire et al. reported that best results with periurethral injections of collagen were obtained in patients with less severe incontinence.[46]

Santarosa and Blaivas reported the results of periurethral fat injections in six men with postprostatectomy incontinence.[47] Mean follow-up was 18 months. None of the patients were dry. Four patients had some modest improvement for 4 to 6 weeks following injection and two patients showed no significant improvement despite repeated injections.

RECONSTRUCTIVE SURGERY

Before the AUS became available, numerous surgical procedures were utilized to restore urinary continence in men. The Young Dees operation creates a long neourethra from the trigone and bladder base associated with ureteral reimplantation.[48] This operation is indicated to correct urinary incontinence associated with epispadias. The anterior tube reconstruction, described by Tanagho, uses the anterior bladder wall to create a tubularized

TABLE 6.5. Results of Collagen Injections to Treat Postprostatectomy Incontinence

	Dry (%)	Improved (%)	Failure (%)	Follow-up (months)	Number of injections	Volume of injection (cc)
Gill[45] (n = 17)	1 (6)	8 (47)	8 (47)	3	2.3	23
Liu[44] (n = 20)	2 (10)	10 (50)	8 (40)	5	2	22
Stothers[37] (n = 10)	1 (10)	3 (30)	6 (60)	6	NA	NA
McGuire[40] (n = 134)	22 (16)	70 (52)	42 (32)	12	NA	NA
Kageyama[41] (n = 10)	1 (10)	4 (40)	5 (50)	14	1.5	20

NA = not available.

hopefully continent proximal urethra.[49] This procedure has been used to address incontinence associated with trauma, epispadias, and for postprostatectomy incontinence with a reported success rate of 70%.[50]

CONCLUSION

The AUS is the gold standard to correct urinary incontinence caused by sphincteric insufficiency in males, with socially acceptable continence in 90% to 95% of properly selected patients. Continued improvement of the device has rendered the procedure safe and reliable. Conversely, periurethral injections, regardless of the substance injected, have disappointing results.

REFERENCES

1. Turner-Warwick R: The sphincter mechanisms: their relation to prostatic enlargement and its treatment. In Hinman F Jr (ed): *Benign Prostatic Hypertrophy.* New York, Springer Verlag, 1983, p 809.
2. Grosling JA, Dixon JS, Lendon RG: The autonomic innervation of the human male and female bladder neck and proximal urethra. *J Urol* 118:302–305, 1977.
3. Myers RP: Male urethral sphincteric anatomy and radical prostatectomy. *Urol Clin North Am* 18:211–227, 1991.
4. Mark JL, Light JK: Management of urinary incontinence after prostatectomy with artificial urinary sphincter. *J Urol* 142:302–306, 1989.
5. Walsh PC, Jewett AJ: Radical surgery for prostatic cancer. *Cancer* 45:1906–1911, 1980.
6. Rudy DC, Woodside JR, Jeffrey R, et al: Urodynamic evaluation of incontinence in patients undergoing modified Campbell radical retropubic prostatectomy: a prospective study. *J Urol* 132:708–711, 1984.
7. Fowler FJ Jr, Barry MJ, Lu-Yao G, et al: Patient reported complications and follow up treatment after radical prostatectomy. The national Medicare experience: 1988–1990 (updated June 93). *Urology* 42:622–629, 1993.
8. Fowler FJ Jr, Barry MJ, Lu-Yao G, et al: Effect of radical prostatectomy for prostate cancer on patient quality of life: result from a Medicare survey. *Urology* 45:1007–1015, 1995.
9. Litwin MS, Hays RD, Fink A, et al: Quality of life outcomes in men treated for localized prostate cancer. *JAMA* 273:129–135, 1995.
10. Zimmern PE, Leach GE: Treatment of incontinence in men. *Semin Urol* 7:124–132, 1989.
11. Barbalias GA, Blaivas JG: Neurologic implication of the pathologically open bladder neck. *J Urol* 129:780–782, 1983.
12. Leach GE, Yun SK: Post prostatectomy incontinence, Parts I and II. *Neurourol Urodyn* 11:91–105, 1992.
13. Leach GE, Yip C, Donovan BJ: Post prostatectomy incontinence: the influence of bladder dysfunction. *J Urol* 138:574–578, 1987.
14. Foote J, Yun S, Leach GE: Post prostatectomy incontinence: pathophysiology, evaluation and management. *Urol Clin North Am* 18:229–241, 1991.
15. Chao R, Mayo ME: Incontinence after radical prostatectomy: detrusor or sphincter causes. *J Urol* 154:16–18, 1995.

16. Goluboff ET, Chang DT, Olsson CA, et al: Urodynamics and the etiology of post prostatectomy urinary incontinence: the initial Columbia experience. *J Urol* 153:1034–1037, 1995.

17. Leach GL, Trockman B, Wong A, et al: Post prostatectomy incontinence: 10 year experience with 215 men. *J Urology* (In press).

18. Leach GE, Raz S: Perfusion sphincterometry: method of intraoperative evaluation of artificial urinary sphincter function. *Urology* 21:212–215, 1983.

19. Fishmann IJ, Shabsigh R, Scott FB: Experience with the artificial urinary sphincter model AS 800 in 148 patients. *J Urol* 141:307–312, 1989.

20. Perez LM, Webster GD: Successful outcome of artificial urinary sphincter in men with post prostatectomy urinary incontinence despite adverse implantation features. *J Urol* 148:1166–1170, 1992.

21. Leo ME, Barrett DM: Success of the narrow-backed cuff design of the AMS 800 artificial urinary sphincter. Analysis of 144 patients. *J Urol* 150:1412–1414, 1993.

22. Light JK, Reynolds JC: Impact of the new cuff design on reliability of the AS 800 artifical urinary sphincter. *J Urol* 147:609–611, 1992.

23. Montague DK: The artificial urinary sphincter (AS 800): experience in 166 consecutive patients. *J Urol* 147:380–382, 1992.

24. Gundian JC, Barrett DM, Parulkar BG: Mayo Clinic experience with the AS 800 artificial urinary sphincter for urinary incontinence after transurethral resection of prostate or open prostatectomy. *Urology* 41:318–321, 1993.

25. Wang Y, Hadley HR: Experience with the artificial sphincter in irradiated patients. *J Urol* 147:612–613, 1992.

26. Barrett DM, Furlow WL: Artificial urinary sphincter in children. In Kelalis PP, King LR, Belman B (eds): *Clinical Pediatric Urology,* vol 1, ed 2. Philadelphia, WB Saunders, 1985.

27. Furlow WF, Barrett DM: Recurrent or persistent urinary incontinence in patients with the artificial urinary sphincter. Diagnostic considerations and management. *J Urol* 133:792–795, 1985.

28. Leach GE: Incontinence after artificial urinary sphincter placement. *J Urol* 138:529–532, 1987.

29. Lang G, Hadley HR, Salter H: Artificial urinary sphincter: the role of ultrasonography in the patient with persistent or recurrent incontinence. *J Urol* 151:325A, 1994.

30. Ghoneim GM, Lapeyrolerie J, Sood OP, et al: Tulane experience with management of urinary incontinence after placement of an artificial urinary sphincter. *World J Urol* 12:333–336, 1994.

31. Kreder KJ, Webster GD: Evaluation and management of incontinence after implantation of the urinary sphincter. *Urol Clin North AM* 18:375–381, 1991.

32. Martins FE, Boyd SD: Artificial urinary sphincter in patients following major pelvic surgery and/or radiotherapy: are they less favorable candidates? *J Urol* 153:1188–1191, 1995.

33. Brito G, Mulcahy JJ, Mitchell ME, et al: Use of a double cuff AMS 800 urinary sphincter for severe stress urinary incontinence. *U Urol* 149:283–285, 1993.

34. Politano VA, Small MP, Harper JM, et al: Periurethral teflon injection for urinary incontinence. *J Urol* 111:379–382, 1974.

35. Claes H, Stoobauts D, Van Meerbeek J, et al: Pulmonary migration following periurethral polytetrafluorethylene injection for urinary incontinence. *J Urol* 142:821–822, 1989.

36. Appell AR: Collagen injection therapy for urinary incontinence. *Urol Clin North Am* 21:177–186, 1994.

37. Stothers L, Chopra A, Raz S: A cost-effectiveness and utility analysis of the artificial urinary sphincter and collagen injections in the treatment of post prostatectomy incontinence. *J Urol* 153:278A, 1995.

38. Santiago Gonzales de Garibay AS, Castro Morrondo J, Castillo Jimeno JM, et al: Endoscopic injection of autologous adipose tissue in the treatment of female incontinence. *Arch Esp Urol* 42:143–147, 1989.

39. Ganabathi K, Leach GE: Periurethral injection techniques. *Atlas Urol Clin North Am* 2:101–109, 1994.

40. McGuire EJ, Appell RA: Transurethral collagen injection for urinary incontinence. *Urology* 43:413–415, 1994.

41. Kageyama S, Kawabe K, Suzuki K, et al: Collagen implantation for post prostatectomy incontinence: early experience with a transrectal ultrasonographically guided method. *J Urol* 152:1473–1475, 1994.

42. Kabalin JN: Treatment of post prostatectomy stress urinary incontinence with periurethral polytetrafluoroethylene paste injection. *J Urol* 152:1463–1466, 1994.

43. Politano VA: Transurethral polytef injection for post prostatectomy urinary incontinence. *Br J Urol* 69:26–28, 1992.

44. Liu J, Flood HD: Selection of patients with intrinsic sphincteric deficiency for treatment with collagen: can we do better? *J Urol* 153:277A, 1995.

45. Gill HS, Payne CK: Experience with collagen injection therapy in men with urinary incontinence. *J Urol* 153:277A, 1995.

46. McGuire EJ, O'Connell HE, Aboseif SR, et al: Collagen injection therapy in treatment of incontinence secondary to radical retropubic prostatectomy. Presented at the Urodynamic Society, Las Vegas, 1995.

47. Santarosa RP, Blaivas JG: Periurethral injection of autologous fat for the treatment of sphincteric incontinence. *J Urol* 151:607–611, 1994.

48. Leadbetter GW Jr: Surgical correction of total urinary incontinence. *J Urol* 91:261–266, 1964.

49. Tanagho EA: Bladder neck reconstruction for total urinary incontinence: 10 years experience. *J Urol* 125:321–326, 1981.

50. Hadley HR, Zimmern PE, Raz S: The treatment of male urinary incontinence. In Walsh PC, Guittes RF, Perlmutter AD (eds): *Campbell's Urology,* ed 5. Philadelphia, WB Saunders, 1986, pp 2658–2678.

7

Surgical Treatment of Detrusor Overactivity

Helen E. O'Connell
Edward J. McGuire
Michael J. Kennelly

INTRODUCTION—THE DETRUSOR AS AN EXPULSIVE FORCE

Definition of Detrusor Overactivity

Urinary leakage as a result of a bladder contraction that is unexpected, uncontrolled, or uncontrollable (motor urge incontinence) has been subdivided by the International Continence Society into two subtypes called *detrusor instability* and *detrusor hyperreflexia*. *Detrusor instability* is present when the detrusor objectively contracts spontaneously or on provocation during the filling phase of a cystometrogram (CMG) while the patient is attempting to inhibit micturition.[1] The term *hyperreflexia* designates the same urodynamic findings but does so in the presence of objective evidence of a relevant neurologic disorder. Ambulatory urodynamic monitoring has demonstrated repeatedly that a CMG will detect only a portion of patients who have motor urge incontinence, i.e., the CMG is not a particularly sensitive test for excluding detrusor contractility as the cause of incontinence.[2,3] In addition, some patients who have detrusor instability on the basis of a CMG are completely continent. These discrepancies make the clinical and urodynamic definition of motor urge incontinence difficult. Clearly, it is inappropriate to exclude as many as 40–50% of people who have a detrusor contraction as the cause of their incontinence on the basis of a CMG.[2,3] It is equally impractical to insist that all patients with urge incontinence must have ambulatory urodynamics to prove that detrusor overactivity is the cause of their symptoms, quite apart from the fact that ambulatory urodynamics has not been studied as to specificity or sensitivity.

The best results of treatment for patients with detrusor contractile incontinence due to detrusor overactivity depend on the identification and elimination of causative or associated conditions such as bladder outlet obstruction and stress incontinence (due to either intrinsic sphincter deficiency or urethral hypermobility). Treatment directed at the detrusor without treatment of the underlying condition almost always fails. When there is no evidence of these underlying disorders, motor urge incontinence is regarded as idiopathic.

Stress Incontinence (Incontinence Due to Urethral Dysfunction)

Some 32% of women with stress incontinence will also have detrusor instability (associated with positive CMG findings).[4] If the stress incontinence is treated, in two-thirds the detrusor instability will resolve, but in one-third it will remain. Thus, in this fairly large group of women suffering from detrusor instability evaluation of urethral function by physical examination, abdominal leak point pressure testing (preferably guided by fluoroscopy) is important. This kind of testing can exclude the condition stress incontinence.[5] In other words, urodynamic assessment of urethral sphincter function is more accurate and sensitive than urodynamic assessment of the detrusor contractile control mechanism. Patients with mixed symptoms should be tested for urethral dysfunction, since that condition frequently is associated with urge incontinence symptoms. If stress incontinence is present it can be characterized as either intrinsic sphincter deficiency, urethral hypermobility, or a combination of these. There are no prospective studies which suggest that in the presence of significant urethral sphincter dysfunction, treatment of motor urge incontinence will completely resolve symptoms. What data is available suggests that treatment is best, first directed at the stress incontinence. When detrusor instability persists after effective treatment of stress incontinence, that condition can be treated as a primary problem. Genital prolapse identification and characterization is also very important in that these conditions may be responsible for detrusor overactivity as well as poor bladder emptying.

Bladder Outlet Obstruction

Bladder outlet obstruction is often associated with detrusor instability. This may be due to benign prostatic hyperplasia, congenital bladder neck obstruction or may follow urethral surgery, e.g., for stress incontinence. When bladder outlet obstruction is shown to coexist with detrusor instability, relief of obstruction, e.g., bladder neck incision, transurethral resection of the prostate,[6] or in women, urethrolysis usually results in the resolution of the underlying detrusor abnormality.[7] In the very elderly, however, total resolution of underlying detrusor instability is much less common.

Motor urge incontinence does not have any relationship to detrusor strength and can coexist with poor contractility. When these conditions coexist the syndrome has been called detrusor hyperactivity with impaired detrusor contractility.[9] Treatment of symptomatic detrusor overactivity may exacerbate a tendency to poor bladder emptying necessitating intermittent catheterization.

Patterns of Idiopathic Motor Urge Incontinence and Their Treatment

In the elderly, the pattern of urge incontinence is often random with the intervals between incontinent episodes being unrelated to bladder volume or the time since last voiding.[10] This pattern of detrusor contractility appears to be due to a poor detrusor warning and control system. The CMG in these patients is typically "normal." Anticholinergic medication is not very effective and behavioral modification such as timed voiding in addition to low-dose anticholinergic medication seem to yield the best outcome. An Ingleman-Sundberg transvaginal denervation procedure in this setting in women may reduce the severity of the motor urge incontinence and make anticholinergic medication unnecessary or more effective.

When the CMG is positive for an uncontrollable contraction, the bladder usually responds to anticholinergic treatment in a predictable fashion. Treatment is directed at lowering bladder pressure, decreasing the frequency of involuntary detrusor contractions by increasing the volumes at which these occur. Therapy may not always result in "complete" continence, but a bladder response can almost always be documented. In patients with an underlying neurologic disorder there is a high probability that intermittent catheterization will be required in conjunction with anticholinergic medication. When incontinence or elevated bladder pressures are still a problem despite anticholinergic therapy and timed emptying, surgical treatment to enlarge the bladder is the next step. Factors such as the age and general condition of the patient, the magnitude of the surgery being considered, and the nature of the underlying disorder determine the appropriateness of a given surgical strategy.

Low Bladder Compliance

Lower urinary tract storage disorders include detrusor reflex overactivity and low bladder compliance. Bladder compliance is reliably evaluated by a CMG. During the filling phase of a CMG, an increase in pressure in response to filling reflects low bladder compliance. Low compliance has considerable prognostic significance and its identification with a CMG is extremely valuable. This was first noted in myelodysplastic patients, where the significance of low bladder compliance with respect to the upper tract function was reported in the early 1980s.[11] In a group of patients with poorly compliant bladders characterized by urethral leakage at detrusor pressures greater than 40 cm H_2O, the tendency to upper tract deterioration was prospectively found to be 100%.[12] Longitudinal studies of myelodysplastic patients indicate that periodic monitoring of detrusor storage and leak point pressures permits the detection of those patients at risk for upper track deterioration. Bladder pressure monitoring is much more effective than radiologic monitoring at the early detection of a risk to upper tract.[13]

Low bladder compliance is most frequently associated with neurologic conditions, but other conditions such as bladder outlet obstruction, posterior urethral valves, an artificial urinary sphincter, pelvic radiation, radical pelvic surgery, cystitis (interstitial, tuberculous, drug-induced), carcinoma in situ or its treatment, e.g., bacillus Calmette-Guérin (BCG) or mitomycin therapy, and longstanding catheterization may also be causative.

Compliance abnormalities seem to be associated with gradual fibrosis of the detrusor.[14] However, in some circumstances low compliance may be reversible, e.g., a child with myelodysplasia, managed by intermittent catheterization. This occurs when despite intermittent catheterization and anticholinergic medication in a myelodysplastic patient, the detrusor pressure at the time of urethral leakage is greater than 40 cm H_2O. In this situation, if external sphincter dilatation is performed and the leak point detrusor pressure reduced to 20 or less, bladder compliance has been shown to dramatically improve without any effect on continence.[15] Sphincterotomy has a similar effect on bladder compliance in paraplegic males, provided the detrusor leak point pressure is made suitably low. These observations suggest that in some circumstances low compliance is reversible, and further that it is the interaction between outlet resistance and the detrusor which seems to lead to low compliance rather than some other inexorable process, due to an underlying neurologic lesion. Although poorly understood, this detrusor–urethral interaction can be seen in other situations e.g., the implantation of an artificial urinary sphincter or benign prostatic hyperplasia with bladder outlet obstruction, both of which can result in a gradual deterioration in bladder compliance.[16,17]

If treatment is instigated before the development of fibrosis, low compliance may be cured and ultimately fibrosis avoided.[18] In the presence of significant fibrosis, surgery such as augmentation cystoplasty may be the only method to restore safe reservoir function.[19]

Dual Treatment Goals—Decrease Detrusor Pressure and Improve Continence

Serious sequelae of elevated bladder storage pressures include vesicoureteral reflux, hydroureteronephrosis and renal parenchymal loss, febrile urinary tract infections, stone formation, renal impairment, and ultimately endstage renal failure. The most critical treatment goal is maintenance of low-pressure bladder urine storage, i.e., normal bladder reservoir function. A secondary effect of improved reservoir function is improved continence. In some circumstances, e.g., idiopathic motor urge incontinence with normal emptying function, the goal of treatment may be purely to improve continence.

HISTORICAL PROCEDURES

Denervation Procedures

Peripheral Denervation Techniques

In 1952, Ingelman-Sundberg described a partial bladder denervation procedure to treat motor urge incontinence[20] particularly when anticholinergic medication was ineffective. A primary cure rate of 88% was reported with a recurrence rate of 11%. The operation was observed to be "quick and easy" after "one has learned how to locate the plexus." Variations on this procedure included the use of phenol to block the same plexus either transvaginally or transvesically.[20,21]

Phenolization

Phenol and other chemicals have been used to cause denervation at a number of sites including the sacral roots[22] and the pelvic plexus,[23,24] the latter being administered either transvaginally or transvesically. When injected into selected sacral roots, good initial results and minimal morbidity were reported for periods of 4 months to 2 years.[22] Long-term results with these procedures were not good, and chemical rhizotomy was later found to be ineffective at permanently abolishing detrusor overactivity.[28]

Similarly, the use of phenol injection to block the pelvic plexus has fallen from favor. Regardless of the route of application, results varied enormously from 75% cure rate to "no significant objective change in any urodynamic parameter in the group as a whole."[27] In addition, significant morbidity was associated with transvaginal or transvesical injection including vesicovaginal fistula,[24,25] rectovaginal fistula, and temporary sciatic nerve palsy.[26]

Cystolysis, Cystocystoplasty, and Bladder Transection

Cystolysis and cystocystoplasty were procedures described by Turner-Warwick to denervate the bladder. These were used for the unstable bladder[33] and interstitial cystitis.[34] These procedures involved open surgical division of nerves supplying the bladder by extensive mobilization of the bladder. Mundy's modification, which involved the division of perivesical tissue and bladder transection, was associated with a 78% cure rate for incontinence at 12 months.[35] Nine of the 23 patients were urodynamically evaluated and either a normal CMG or a "shift to the right" was demonstrated.

With the aim of decreasing the magnitude of the procedure, particularly the need for a large abdominal incision, Parsons[36] used an endoscopic transection technique, reporting an 82% improvement rate. A subsequent series,[37] however, found that out of 18 patients, 14 were unchanged and only 2 rendered continent. With the increasing use of augmentation cystoplasty, which yielded a considerably more reliable relief of urge incontinence, the popularity of these procedures ceased.

Complete and Selective Sacral Rhizotomy

The division of both anterior and posterior rootlets of S1–S5, referred to as complete rhizotomy, was performed with the aim of abolishing reflex bladder activity in spinal cord injured patients. This particularly applied to women in whom sphincterotomy is not an option. Men were generally not considered suitable for rhizotomy because of a concern about loss of sexual function. None of the literature in this area indicates the effect of such procedures on sexual function in women. Complete sacral rhizotomy often leads to detrusor hypertonicity and recurrent incontinence on that basis. Transection of the sacral dorsal roots only, was found to be much more effective with regard to detrusor contractility and was not associated with hypertonicity of the detrusor.[28] These procedures have been used in conjunction with intermittent catheterization, or with anterior root stimulators to induce bladder emptying.

In patients with idiopathic enuresis, multiple sclerosis, myelodysplasia, and spinal cord injury, division of S3 sacral nerves, either unilaterally or bilaterally has also been performed.[29] Mixed results were obtained with a good to very good early response noted in seven of nine patients. Upper tract deterioration later occurred, and the effects on continence were often short-lived.

Hydrodistention

Hydrostatic bladder distention was originally described for the treatment of bladder tumors[30] and currently is a treatment for patients with interstitial cystitis. It has also been used with mixed efficacy in the treatment of motor urge incontinence. In the experimental setting, overdistention has been found to cause degeneration of unmyelinated motor and sensory nerve fibers.[32] Success rates varied from 18% to 77% although complications were not uncommon with bladder perforation occurring in as many as 8% of cases. Moreover, long-term results for idiopathic or hyperreflexic detrusor contractility were so poor that the procedure was abandoned.

CURRENT SURGICAL MANAGEMENT

Neural Modulation

Intradural neural modulation techniques may be used to decrease detrusor overactivity and modify other vesicourethral dysfunctions[38] in paralyzed patients. Evolved from the work of Brindley,[40] direct sacral root stimulation with a neurosurgically implanted electrode is currently in use in European centers. The nerve roots are identified using an operating microscope and urodynamic testing is performed simultaneously. The anterior root can be distinguished from the posterior root by its color, position, and size, and stimulation is used to confirm the effect of nerve root division. The dorsal roots of S1 through S4 are divided and coagulated. A sacral anterior root stimulator may then be used of effect voiding after the deafferentation results in abolition of reflex activity.

Noll reported a series of 162 patients with refractory detrusor hyperactivity treated with intradural stimulation after sacral root deafferentation. At a mean of 2.5 years followup, 95% were continent with an areflexic bladder.[38] Those who were incontinent had previously had sphincteric surgical procedures performed. Deafferentation in conjunction with an anterior root stimulator also resulted in an abolition of autonomic dysreflexia in 89 of the 101 cases. Improvement in renal function, vesicoureteral reflux, and febrile urinary tract infection accompanied these changes.

These results are significantly better than those reported previously which Noll attributed to the completeness of the deafferentation in the more recent series. Suitable candidates for intradural stimulation are patients with refractory detrusor overactivity despite maximal anticholinergic medication and intermittent catheterization. Whether this type of therapy would be acceptable for a non-neurogenic population with debilitating motor urge incontinence remains to be seen.

Schmidt used percutaneous testing of sacral nerve root stimulation to gauge whether useful responses could be obtained by implantation of an extradural or intradural stimulator without routine deafferentation.[39] Stimulation has been used for voiding dysfunction, urge and stress incontinence, and pelvic pain syndromes in non spinal cord injured patients, as well as deafferentation and root stimulation in spinal cord injured patients.[41]

Modified Ingelman-Sundberg Denervation Procedure

The Ingelman-Sundberg procedure as described in 1952 and 1959 involved a relatively extensive denervation procedure via a vaginal incision.[21] A modified version of the procedure to reduce its magnitude resulted in very few complications and a 75% rate of cure or significant improvement.[42] A local anesthetic block is used to test whether temporary denervation results in a complete resolution of symptoms. To do this 10 cc of 0.5% bupivicaine is injected via a 23-gauge spinal needle into the anterior vaginal wall overlying the trigone. Over the 8–12 hr after the injection, patients observe the effect of the injection. If there is a dramatic reduction in urge incontinence, patients are offered a modified Ingelman-Sundberg procedure.

The procedure is performed under anesthesia, either general or regional. A Foley catheter and self-retaining vaginal speculum are placed to provide access to anterior vaginal wall and the bladder base. Normal saline is injected into the anterior vaginal wall to facilitate the dissection and an inverted "smile" incision is made at the vesicourethral junction, palpated by pulling the catheter snugly against the bladder neck. The vaginal epithelium and perivesical fascia are dissected off the underlying bladder. The dissection is extended in a superior-lateral direction into the limits of the incision to where the terminal branches of the pelvic ganglia and postganglionic fibers lie. Spreading the scissors in this place divides these fibers, resulting in a variable degree of denervation.

This procedure is useful for motor urge incontinence including some women with CMG-negative motor urge incontinence.[42] It is *not* effective, however, for sensory disorders of the bladder such as interstitial cystitis, nor for compliance abnormalities. In properly selective patients, the procedure at one year is associated with clinical dryness (cure) in 64% to 70% of patients. The lower figure is from unpublished, current, University of Texas-Houston data.

Augmentation Cystoplasty

Urinary reconstruction procedures such as augmentation cystoplasty and detrusor mymectomy are treatments used for patients fit enough for abdominal surgery who have disabling detrusor overactivity refractory to conservative therapy. Bladder augmentation makes unstable detrusor contractions ineffectual and/or raises the volume threshold at which they occur. Initially, this condition was treated with supratrigonal cystectomy and augmentation cecocystoplasty. Subsequently the bladder was kept in situ and divided either sagitally[44] or transversely as a "clam"[45] or large bladder flap.[43] Satisfactory results have been reported in 69–97% of patients.[44–48]

While nearly all segments of the gastrointestinal tract have been used for augmentation enterocystoplasty, the ileum is the most popular segment because of its familiarity to the urologist, favorable urodynamic properties when detubularized, a decrease in anastomotic complications where the bowel continuity is restored relative to colonic anastomoses, and the ease with which it is mobilized for an anastomosis to the bladder.[49] The metabolic complications are well known and although they can be severe, methods of management of these complications, including their prevention are well established.

Technique

There are several ways of performing augmentation cystoplasty. Our standard technique, which would be modified depending upon which bowel segment seemed most appropriate for use at the time of laparotomy and whether additional procedures such as bladder neck closure or an appendiceal stoma were indicated, is described.

All patients undergo a bowel preparation. Through a midline incision, the bladder and terminal ileum are exposed and a large anteriorly based bladder flap is created. A suitable 20- to 25-cm segment of ileum 10–15 cm proximal to the ileocecal valve is selected. A stapled ileal end-to-end anastomosis is performed to restore bowel continuity (Fig. 7.1A). The ileal segment is detubularized along its antimesenteric border leaving the distal 1 cm ends intact. The ileal segment is folded upon itself in the shape of a "U" (Fig. 7.1B). The backwall unites the two arms of the individual bowel segments is hand-sewn with a continuous single layer of chromic catgut suture. The detubularized bowel is anastomosed to the wide open mouth of the bladder flap (Fig. 7.1C). A suprapubic tube and urethral catheter are placed before closure to drain the augmentation for 10–14 days.

Using the technique, in 69 patients with uncontrollable motor urge incontinence and/or detrusor hyperreflexia a 93% rate of cure of incontinence was achieved. Of the failures, four had low pressure reflex detrusor activity associated with a reflexly mediated fall in intrinsic sphincter pressure and stress incontinence.

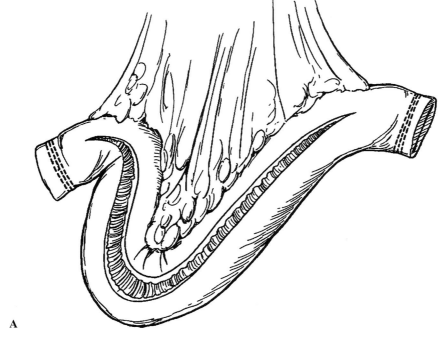

A

Fig. 7.1A: Small bowel segment is isolated and opened along the antimesenteric border. Typically the length is 25 cms.

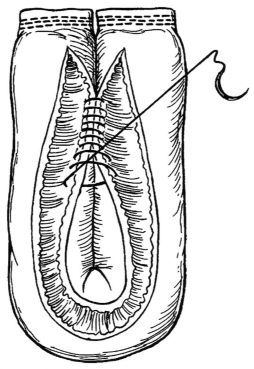

B

Fig. 7.1B: Closure of the posterior reservoir wall with a running suture. This will be followed by partial closure of the anterior wall involving the upper 1/3 of the opening.

129

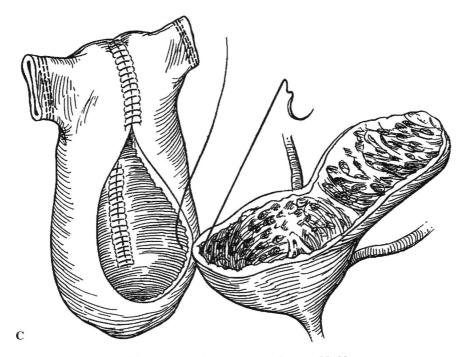

Fig. 7.1C: Anastomosis of the augmentation segment to the open bladder.

Complications from augmentation cystoplasty included those related to intra-abdominal surgery such as adhesive small bowel obstruction and wound-related complications. The major complications related specifically to the augmentation include bladder or augmentation segment calculi, augmentation perforation, and the need to perform lifelong intermittent catheterization in a high proportion of patients.[47] In order to cope with intermittent catheterization, patients need to be motivated and have reasonable manual dexterity.

Detrusor Mymectomy (Bladder Autoaugmentation)

The significant morbidity associated with augmentation cystoplasty encouraged the development of alternative bladder augmentation procedures. In 1989, Cartwright and Snow performed the first bladder autoaugmentations in seven pediatric patients with neurovesical dysfunction.[50] This extraperitoneal procedure involves the meticulous excision of a cap of detrusor muscle keeping intact the underlying mucosa. This procedure obviates the use of bowel, avoiding the development of the majority of augmentation cystoplasty complications. The operative time and duration of hospitalization (40–100 min and 3–5 days respectively) are considerably less than the requirements for augmentation cystoplasty.

Prior to the operation, a Foley catheter is placed and connected to an irrigating set to permit filling and emptying of the bladder throughout the procedure. Via a Pfannenstiel incision the bladder is exposed. An incision is made in the detrusor musculature with a scalpel until the bladder mucosa protrudes. The detrusor muscle is sharply dissected off the anterior, lateral, and superior surfaces of the bladder. Filamentous bands of detrusor muscle are left intact. The bladder is repeatedly filled and emptied to facilitate dissection.

While extreme care is used to avoid penetrating the mucosa during this dissection, if a mucosal hole occurs, it is closed with a 4-0 chromic suture. We do not drain the prevesical space and the Foley catheter is removed as early as the first postoperative day. Intermittent catheterization is instituted as soon as the catheter is removed. Patients with neurogenic conditions do not void, while 80% of those with a normal bladder contraction preoperatively are voiding well by 4 weeks, and virtually all are voiding by 3 months. Patients with impaired detrusor function (i.e., radiation cystitis) usually require intermittent catheterization, but not always.

Swami et al. treated 32 patients with intractable detrusor overactivity with detrusor mymectomy with an 88% success rate in relieving symptoms and a 78% continent rate.[51] Postoperative urodynamics showed a significant increases in bladder capacity and improvement in bladder compliance. Some patients exhibit persistent detrusor reflex activity that is usually low-amplitude and occurs at larger than normal volumes. In children, Cartwright and Snow reserve the procedure for the treatment of refractory poor compliance when the bladder capacity is at least 75% of expected capacity for age. In those with more severe restrictions, augmentation ileocystoplasty is performed from the outset.[52] The short-term results from detrusor mymectomy for detrusor overactivity are encouraging although further evaluation is clearly required to establish its long-term merit.

Ileovesicostomy

When hand function is inadequate for intermittent catheterization, in patients with detrusor overactivity resulting in incapacitating incontinence or upper tract deterioration, an incontinent ileovesicostomy provides low pressure drainage and is an effective long-term solution[53] as distinct from the long-term prognosis that accompanies ileal conduit diversion.[54]

Conclusions

Motor urge incontinence may be associated with or due to stress incontinence, genital prolapse, bladder outlet obstruction, or an underlying neurologic disorder. The latter form of hyperactivity is referred to as detrusor hyperreflexia. Often though, motor urge incontinence is idiopathic. When disabling motor urge incontinence persists despite treatment of the underlying cause, medication and behavioral strategies may be insufficient to reduce leakage and surgical management may be considered. In detrusor hyperreflexia and low bladder compliance the added potential for upper tract deterioration may mandate surgical treatment in order to reduce dangerous bladder pressure refractory to medication and intermittent catheterization.

Useful surgical techniques include the Ingleman-Sundberg procedure to treat motor urge incontinence regardless of whether or not the CMG is positive, intradural deafferentation, and augmentation procedures. Although intradural stimulation techniques appear to be effective, their availability is restricted and they abolish reflex bladder activity at the expense of reflex erectile activity. A multitude of other denervation procedures have been attempted over the years but only a few have stood the test of time. The treatment of detrusor overactivity is usually associated with the risk of incomplete bladder emptying or the need to perform intermittent catheterization. Augmentation cystoplasty has been used effectively in many centers to improve continence and upper tract function and although it is not without risk, the risks are well known and strategies to minimize them are well established.

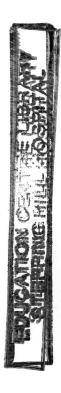

REFERENCES

1. Abrams P, Blaivas PG, Stanton SL, et al: Standardization of terminology of lower urinary tract function. *Neurourol Urodyn* 7:403–427, 1988.

2. Webb RJ, Ramsden PD, Neal DE: Ambulatory monitoring and electronic measurement of urinary leakage in the diagnosis of motor urge incontinence. *Br J Urol* 68:148, 1991.

3. O'Donnell PD, Hanish HM: Telemetric electromyographic monitoring in elderly incontinent men. *Neurourol Urodyn* 11:115–121, 1992.

4. McGuire EJ, Lytton B, Pepe V, et al: Stress urinary incontinence. *Obstet Gynecol* 47:255–264, 1976.

5. McGuire EJ, Fitzpatrick CC, Wan J, et al: Clinical assessment of urethral sphincter function. *J Urol* 150:1452–1454, 1993.

6. Abrams PH: Motor urge incontinence and bladder outlet obstruction. *Neurourol Urodyn* 4:317–328, 1985.

7. Foster HE, McGuire EJ: Management of urethral obstruction with transvaginal urethrolysis. *J Urol* 150:1448, 1993.

8. Gormley EA, Griffiths DJ, McCracken PN, et al: Effect of transurethral resection of the prostate on detrusor instability and urge incontinence in elderly males. *Neurourol Urodyn* 12:445, 1993.

9. Resnick NM, Yalla SV: Detrusor hyperactivity with impaired contractile function: an unrecognized but common cause of incontinence in elderly patients. *JAMA* 257:3076, 1987.

10. O'Donnell PD: The pathophysiology of incontinence in the elderly. *Adv Urol* 4:129, 1991.

11. McGuire EJ, Woodside JR, Borden TA, et al: Prognostic value of urodynamic testing in myelodysplastic patients. *J Urol* 126:205, 1981.

12. McGuire EJ, Woodside JR, Borden TA: Upper urinary tract deterioration in patients with myelodysplasia and detrusor hypertonia: a follow-up study. *J Urol* 129:823, 1983.

13. Kaufman AM, Roberts AC, Rudy DC, et al: Decreased bladder complication in myelomeningocele patients managed by radiologic observation. *J Urol* 153:278A, Abstract 199, 1995.

14. Woodside JR, McGuire EJ: Detrusor hypertonicity as a late complication of a Wertheim hysterectomy. *J Urol* 127:1143–1145, 1982.

15. Wang SC, McGuire EJ, Bloom DA: Urethral dilation in the management of urological complications of myelodysplasia. *J Urol* 142:1054, 1989.

16. Roth D, Dyas PR, Kroovand RL, et al: Urinary tract deterioration associated with the artificial urinary sphincter. *J Urol* 135:94–97, 1986.

17. Light JK, Pietro T: Alteration in detrusor behavior and the effect on renal function following insertion of the artificial urinary sphincter. *J Urol* 136:632–635, 1986.

18. Wang SC, McGuire EJ, Bloom DA: A bladder pressure management system for myelodysplasia—clinical outcome. *J Urol* 140:1499, 1988.

19. Steinberg R, Bennett C, Konnak J, et al: Construction of a low pressure reservoir and achievement of continence after "diversion" and in end stage vesical dysfunction.

20. Ingelman-Sundberg A: Urinary incontinence in women, excluding fistulae. *Acta Obstet Gynecol Scand* 31:266, 1952.

21. Ingleman-Sundberg A: Partial denervation of the bladder. A new operation for the treatment of urge incontinence and similar conditions in women. *Acta Obstet Gynecol Scand* 38:487, 1959.

22. Alloussi S, Loew F, Mast GJ, et al: Treatment of motor urge incontinence of the urinary bladder by selective sacral blockade. *Br J Urol* 46:464–467, 1984.

23. Blackford HN, Murrary K, Stephenson TP, et al: Results of transvesical infiltration of the pelvic plexuses with phenol in 116 patients. *Br J Urol* 56:647–649, 1982.

24. Nordling J, Steven K, Meyhoff HH: Subtrigonal phenol injection: lack of effect in the treatment of detrusor instability. *Neurourol Urodynam* 5:449, 1986.

25. Wall LL, Stanton SL: Transvesical phenol injection of pelvic plexuses in females with refractory urge incontinence. *Br J Urol* 63:465, 1989.

26. Cameron-Strange A, Millard RJ: Management of refractory motor urge incontinence by transvesical phenol injection. *Br J Urol* 62:323, 1988.

27. Ramsay IN, Clancy S, Hilton P: Subtrigonal phenol injections in the treatment of idiopathic detrusor instability in the female—a long term urodynamic follow-up. *Br J Urol* 69:363, 1992.

28. McGuire EJ, Savastano JA: Urodynamic findings and clinical status following vesical denervation procedures for control of incontinence. *J Urol* 132:87–88, 1984.

29. Clarke SJ, Forster MC, Thomas DG: Selective sacral neurectomy in the management of urinary incontinence due to detrusor instability. *Br J Urol* 51:510–514, 1979.

30. Helmstein K: Treatment of bladder carcinoma by a hydrostatic pressure technique. *Br J Urol* 44:434, 1972.

31. Dunn M, Smith JC, Ardran GM: Prolonged bladder distension as a treatment of urgency and urge incontinence. *Br J Urol* 46:645–652, 1974.

32. Sehn JT: Anatomic effect of distention therapy in unstable bladder: a new approach *Urology* 11:581, 1978.

33. Turner-Warwick RT, Handley Ashken M: The functional results of partial, subtotal and total cystocystoplasty with special reference to ureterocystoplasty, selective sphincterotomy and cystocystoplasty. *Br J Urol* 39:3–12, 1967.

34. Worth PHL, Turner-Warwick RT: The treatment of interstitial cystitis by cystolysis with observations on cystoplasty. *Br J Urol* 45:65–71, 1973.

35. Mundy AR: Bladder transection for urge incontinence associated with detrusor instability. *Br J Urol* 52:480–483, 1980.

36. Parsons KF, Machin DG, Woolfenden KA, et al: Endoscopic bladder transection for detrusor instability. *Br J Urol* 59:526–528, 1987.

37. Lucas MG, Thomas DG: Endoscopic bladder transection for detrusor instability. *Br J Urol* 59:526–528, 1987.

38. Noll F: Intradural electrostimulation for the treatment of a spastic bladder. *Adv Urol* 8:439–450, 1995.

39. Schmidt R: Neurostimulation in urology. In Krush ED, McGuire EJ (eds): *Female Urology* Philadelphia, Lippincott, 1994, p 135.

40. Brindley GS: An implant to empty the bladder or close the urethra. *J Neurol Neurosurg Psychiatry* 40:358, 1977.

41. Wan J, McGuire EJ, Wang SC, et al: Ingleman-Sundberg denervation for detrusor instability. *J Urol* 145:Abstract 81, 1991.

42. McGuire EJ, Ritchey ML, Wan JH: Surgical therapy of uncontrollable detrusor contractility. In Kursh ED, McGuire EJ (eds): *Female Urology.* Philadelphia, Lippincott, p 119.

43. Bramble RJ: The treatment of enuresis and urge incontinence by enterocystoplasty. *Br J Urol* 54:693–696, 1982.

44. Kockelbergh RC, Tan JBL, Bates CP, et al: Clam enterocystoplasty in general urological practice. *Br J Urol* 68:38–41, 1991.

45. Kay R, Straffon R: Augmentation cystoplasty. *Urol Clin North Am* 13:295, 1986.

46. Mundy AR, Stephenson T: "Clam" ileocystoplasty for the treatment of refractory urge incontinence. *Br J Urol* 57:641–646, 1985.

47. Goldwasser B, Webster GD: Augmentation and substitution enterocystoplasty. *J Urol* 135:215, 1986.

48. Luangkhot R, Peng BCH, Blaivas JG: Ileocystoplasty for the management of the refractory neurogenic bladder: surgical technique and urodynamic findings. *J Urol* 145:1340, 1991.

49. Flood HD, Mulhotra SJ, O'Connell HE, et al: Long Term Results and Complications Using Augmentation Cystoplasty in Reconstructive Urology. *Neurourol Urodyn* 14:297–309, 1995.

50. Cartwright PC, Snow BW: Bladder autoaugmentation: early clinical experience. *J Urol* 142:505, 1989.

51. Swami SK, Abrams P, Hammonds JC, et al: Treatment of detrusor overactivity with detrusor mymectomy (bladder autoaugmentation). Soc Int d'Urol 23rd Congress Abstract 580, 1994.

52. Cartwright PC, Snow BW: Bladder autoaugmentation. *Adv Urol* 8:273, 1995.

53. Schwartz SL, Kennelly MJ, McGuire EJ, et al: Incontinent ileo-vesicostomy urinary diversion in the treatment of lower urinary tract dysfunction. *J Urol* 152:99–102, 1994.

54. Hampel N, Bodner DR, Persky L: Ileal and jejunal conduit urinary diversion. *Urol Clin North Am* 13:207, 1986.

8

Periurethral Injectables for the Treatment of Sphincteric Incontinence in Men and Women

Rodney A. Appell
J. Christian Winters

Urinary incontinence may originate at the level of the bladder or the urethra. In evaluating patients for the use of intraurethral injections as a treatment of urinary incontinence, it is essential to identify the cause of incontinence in order to recommend appropriate therapy. Intraurethral injections benefit patients with incontinence occurring at the level of the urethra. Incontinence occurring at the level of the urethra may be due to anatomic displacement of a normally functioning urethra (urethral hypermobility) in females or intrinsic incompetence of the urethral closure mechanism (intrinsic sphincteric dysfunction) in females or males. Patients with intrinsic sphincteric dysfunction (ISD) commonly have had a previous surgical procedure on or near the urethra, a sympathetic neurologic injury, or myelodysplasia. In female patients with hypermobility of the bladder neck and proximal urethra the condition results from a deficiency in pelvic support. These patients benefit from a bladder neck elevation and stabilization. Patients with ISD have poor urethral function and require procedures to increase outflow resistance. Bladder neck suspension procedures will fail in these patients due to the poor urethral function, and these patients require pubovaginal sling procedures, artificial urinary sphincters, or periurethral injections.

In patients with ISD, the presence or absence of anatomic support will assist in directing future management. At present, patients with a lack of anatomic support (hypermobility) and ISD do best undergoing sling procedures or artificial urinary sphincters. Patients

135

with a fixed, well-supported urethra in association with ISD are excellent candidates for periurethral injection. During the multicenter investigation of collagen in the treatment of ISD, the patients selected with incontinence due to hypermobility (Type II) did not fair well.[1,2] Therefore, the recommendation currently is to perform intraurethral or periurethral injections on patients with a poorly functioning urethra (ISD) and good anatomic support. However, recent data suggest that intraurethral injections may be used for selected patients with Type II stress urinary incontinence.[3]

EVALUATION AND PATIENT SELECTION

When obtaining a history from patients with urinary incontinence, it is important to elucidate if previous surgery has been performed or an underlying neurologic disorder exists. Also, the activity precipitating urinary leakage is important. Patients who leak in the supine position, have bedwetting, or leak with a sensation of urinary urgency often do not have genuine stress urinary incontinence and need to be investigated for bladder and/or intrinsic sphincteric deficiency. In women, the physical examination is essential to ascertain if concomitant urogenital prolapse and urethral hypermobility are present. The Q-tip test is useful for diagnosing urethral hypermobility (UH).[4] An angle of greater than 30° signifies UH.

Urodynamic studies are performed to evaluate possible bladder causes of incontinence (instability, decreased contractility/overflow) and to evaluate urethral function. Tests of urethral function may be performed using leak point pressures or urethral pressure profiles. The Valsalva leak point pressure (VLPP) is the vesical pressure required to drive urine through the urethra. This corresponds to urethral opening pressure and low urethral opening pressure implies minimal urethral resistance and poor urethral function. Therefore, leakage per urethra in patients with ISD occurs at low abdominal leak point pressures. The VLPP is obtained by filling the bladder and asking the patient to strain, at incremental bladder volumes of 50 ml beginning at 150 ml and followed to 300 ml. The pressure is recorded at which urine leaks through the urethra. Leakage can be identified either by direct vision or by fluoroscopic assessment of contrast during a videourodynamic procedure. VLPP of less the 60 cm of water signifies poor or absent urethral function. We believe these measurements correlate with urethral pressure profiles and are less variable and easier to perform.[5] Videourodynamics are urodynamic studies performed in conjunction with radiographic analysis of the bladder. The presence of an open bladder neck with the bladder at rest in the absence of a detrusor contraction implies the presence of ISD. Patients who have undergone multiple surgical procedures, have mixed incontinence, or with neurogenic bladders benefit greatly from videourodynamic procedures. The ideal patient for periurethral injections is a patient with poor urethral function, normal bladder capacity, and good anatomic support. A clear advantage of injectables in ISD is the attainment of increased urethral closing function with only minor increases in urethral closing pressure. Patients with minimal hypermobility and high leak point pressure or elderly, less active females with anatomic incontinence may be considered for periurethral injections as well, however it is wise to reserve this therapy for patients in this population who represent a surgical risk or have a more limited mobility.

Contraindications to periurethral injections include active urinary tract infection, untreated detrusor instability, and known hypersensitivity to the injected agent. Patients who are to have intraurethral injection of collagen must undergo skin testing 1 month prior to the procedure to determine if hypersensitivity to the material is present.[6] In the Gax collagen multicenter trial, 4% of the female patients exhibited hypersensitivity during skin testing, where as only 1% of males exhibited hypersensitivity.[7]

INJECTABLE MATERIALS

The ideal material for periurethral injection is one that is easily injected, biocompatible, and causes little or no inflammatory reaction. Also, the substance should elicit no immunogenic response. There should be no migration of the injected material, and it should maintain its bulking effect for a long period of time. Many agents have been used as injectables for urinary incontinence ranging from sclerosing agents to autologous blood.[8,9] Currently, the most widely used agent is crosslinked bovine collagen. Collagen (Contigen) received United States Food and Drug Administration approval for the treatment of ISD in male and female patients in September 1993. Autologous fat has gained acceptance in patients who decline or have demonstrated hypersensitivity to collagen, but it is technically more difficult to inject.[10] Polytetrafluoroethylene (PTFE) paste has recently been removed from the United States marketplace due to concerns over its migration and safety,[11] despite no reports of untoward sequelae in human beings.[12] We believe that since these agents may be injected safely under local anesthesia and have some efficacy in patients with hypermobility,[3] there may be additional potential for them to be used as a first line of therapy in patients with stress incontinence who are considered poor surgical risks for open surgical repairs as well as in healthy individuals with ISD.

PTFE Paste (Urethrin)

This is a sterile mixture of PTFE micropolymer particles, glycerine, and polysorbate. PTFE particles stimulate an ingrowth of fibroblasts at the injection site, become encapsulated and produce a permanent bolstering effect.[12] These particles elicit a chronic foreign body reaction with granuloma formation. Documented evidence of particle migration and granuloma formation have raised concerns about the use of this material.[11]

Autologous Fat

As a periurethral bulking agent, fat has several advantages: it is readily available, biocompatible, and easily obtainable. Fat integrates as a graft, however a significant portion of the injected material is reabsorbed and replaced by inflammation and fibrosis with connective tissue producing the final bulk effect.[10] The technical difficulty with periurethral injection is the major limitation in using fat as an injectable agent. There is no evidence of migration of the injected fat particles.

Glutaraldehyde Crosslinked Bovine Collagen (Contigen)

This agent is both biocompatible and biodegradable. It is a sterile nonpyrogenic bovine dermal collagen crosslinked with glutaraldehyde and dispersed in a phosphate-buffered physiologic saline. The crosslinking process improves the integrity of the material for the injection by increasing its resistance to collagenase as well as decreasing the antigenicity of the collagen. A minimal inflammatory response has been associated with the injection of collagen and no granuloma formation or foreign body reaction is present. Also no foreign body reaction occurs. Contigen begins to degrade in approximately 12 weeks, however, in this period of time neovascularization and the deposition by fibroblasts of host collagen occurs within the implant. The collagen completely degrades within 10–19 months.[13] There are no reports of particle migration of the collagen material.[14]

Silicone Polymers

Macroplastique and Bioplastique consist of textured silicone macroparticles suspended within a hydrogel. The hydrogel is rapidly absorbed by the host tissue, however the macroimplant becomes fixed in position by encapsulation. The particle size is greater than 100 μm which inhibits migration.[15] Henly et al. compared migratory and histologic tendencies of solid silicone macrospheres to smaller silicone particles in dogs.[15] Nuclear imaging revealed small particles dissipated throughout the lung, kidney, brain, and lymph nodes at 4 months. One episode of large particle migration to the lung occurred without associated inflammation; an x-ray analysis confirmed that the particles were silicone. Initial clinical trials demonstrated the potential of this substance for the treatment of ISD and genuine stress incontinence, however migration has been documented to be a problem with even large particle injections and the use of this material will likely be limited in the United States.[16]

TECHNIQUE OF INJECTION

The technique of injection of material is not difficult; however, it is essential to perform precise placement of the material in order to ensure an optimal result. The injection can be performed either suburothelially through a needle placed directly through a cystoscope (transurethral injection) or periurethrally with a spinal needle inserted percutaneously and positioned in the urethral tissues in the suburothelial space observing the manipulation cystoscopically.[17] While transurethral injections are initially easier to perform than the periurethral technique, we feel that the reduction in potential for transurethral bleeding and extravasation of the injectable into the urethral lumen are worth the frustration of involvement with a technique having a steeper learning curve.

Men are injected predominantly by the transurethral approach, and females are injected by either transcystoscopic implantation of a needle into the suburothelium[18] or by placement of a spinal needle inserted percutaneously along the wall of the urethra while observing the delivery of the material directly by urethroscopy.[17] Also, indirect visualization by ultrasound has been described as useful in the precise localization of the injection.[19] Recently, Neal et al.[20] have introduced a technique to facilitate periurethral needle placement utilizing methylene blue mixed with local anesthesia enabling the surgeon to place the implant more accurately. There is certainly a learning curve with any technique chosen which ultimately results in using less injectable material to attain continence. We will describe the technique of injection in males and females employing collagen, as this is currently the most widely used injectable substance. Following this, we will make additional comments concerning the alterations of techniques in the injection of other injectable materials.

Technique of Injection in the Male Patient

The male patient is positioned in the semilithotomy position and 2% lidocaine jelly is placed intraurethrally and left in place 10 min prior to instrumentation. Cystourethroscopy with a zero degree lens is employed. The injectable material is then delivered suburothelially by way of a transcystoscopic injection needle under direct vision. This is performed in a circumferential matter employing four-quadrant needle placements. The needle is advanced suburothelially in four quadrants and the material is injected until a mucosal bleb is created in each quadrant. Gradually, after employing circumferential injection the urethral mucosa coapts in the midline (Fig. 8.1).

In cases of ISD following post radical prostatectomy surgery, a short segment of urethra remains above the external sphincter. If visualization of this urethra is difficult, the needle may be placed at the level of the external sphincter and advanced to ensure deposition of the material proximal to the external sphincter. It is important to note that the material should not be injected directly into the external sphincter as this can cause pudendal nerve spasm.

Injection is more difficult in patients with postradical prostatectomy incontinence resulting from the short segment of urethra above the level of the external sphincter and extensive scarring which usually occurs in this area following surgery. In order to ensure opti-

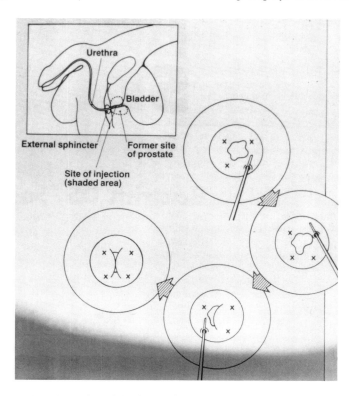

Fig. 8.1. Transurethral circumferential injection in males. From McGuire EJ, Appell RA: Collagen injection for the dysfunctional urethra. *Contemporary Urology* 3:11, 1991. Reproduced with permission.

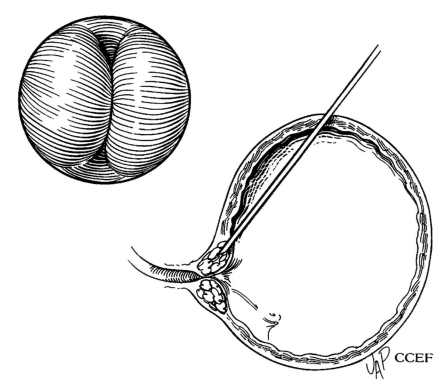

Fig. 8.2. Diagram of antegrade injection.

mal placement of the material proximal to the external sphincter and at the level of the bladder neck, antegrade injections employing either a flexible cystoscope,[21] a small ureteroscope with a 5-Fr working port,[22] or a commercial PTFE injector[23] may be performed through a small suprapubic punch cystotomy. This technique allows more precise localization of the bladder neck and urethra above the level of the external sphincter. In addition, it features injection of the material in more supple, less scarred tissue near the bladder neck (Fig. 8.2). Although only in very early clinical trials, this technique seems to facilitate more precise injection of material generating improved results with the use of less material. (Fig. 8.3). It is the authors' opinion that this technique represents an exciting new method of collagen implantation in the male and should be considered in any male patient not achieving adequate success by way of a transurethral approach.

Technique of Injection in the Female Patient

Women may be injected by way of a transcystoscopic technique[18] or a periurethral approach.[17] The authors prefer the periurethral approach, as this minimizes intraurethral bleeding and extravasation of the injectable substance. With either approach, the woman is placed in the lithotomy position, the introitus is anesthetized with 20% topical benzocaine, and the urethra is anesthetized with topical 2% lidocaine jelly. Following this, a local injection of 1% plain lidocaine is performed periurethrally at the 3 and 9 o'clock positions using 2–4 ml on each side.

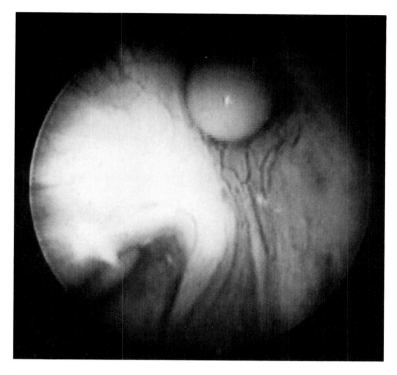

Fig. 8.3. Endoscopic view of antegrade injection.

Panendoscopy is performed with zero or 30° lenses, and a 22-gauge spinal needle with the obturator in place is positioned periurethrally at the 4 or 8 o'clock position with the bevel of the needle directed toward the lumen. The needle is then advanced into the ure-thral muscle in the lamina propria in an entirely suburothelial plane. Once the needle is positioned in the lamina propria it usually advances with very little force. The needle may also be placed at the 6 o'clock position and again needle placement is fully observed endo-scopically. Bulging of the tip of the needle against the lining of the urethra is observed dur-ing advancement of the needle to ensure its proper placement. When the needle tip is prop-erly positioned just below the bladder neck, the material is injected until swelling is visible on each side, creating the appearance of occlusion of the urethral lumen. Once the urethra is approximately 50% occluded, the needle is removed and reinserted on the opposite side and additional material is injected until mucosa coapts in the midline creating the endo-scopic appearance of two lateral prostatic lobes (Fig. 8.4A–C).

The technique and approaches chosen for the injection of PTFE for urinary incontinence are similar to the Contigen injection with the exception of the depth of penetration of the needle. As stated previously, the needle placement for the injection of Contigen is sub-urothelially just behind the urethra mucosa. However, if the needle is placed too superfi-cially for PTFE injection, the material may perforate and extrude into the urethral lumen which can be problematic as the PTFE is sometimes difficult to remove. Therefore, when performing a PTFE injection the needle is inserted as a 45° angle which allows deposition of the material 2 cm below the urethral mucosa.[24] This allows for the adequate bulk-

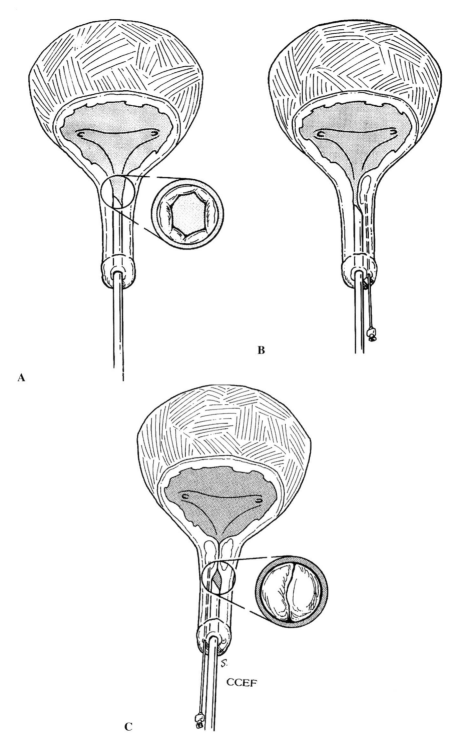

Fig. 8.4. A: Diagram of cytoscopic view of bladder neck prior to injection in the female. **B:** Diagram of periurethral needle placement in the female. **C:** Diagram of completed bladder neck coaptation during periurethral injection in the famale.

enhancing effect minimizing the possibility of a perforation and extrusion of the injected Teflon into the urethra.

The technique of injection of autologous fat is divided into two phases: (1) harvesting the fat, and (2) periurethral injection of the fat. There are multiple variations in the technique to harvest autologous fat, ranging from aspiration with a large bore needle to liposuction.[25,26] The authors use the Tulip fat harvesting and injection system to obtain autologous fat. An injection cannula is used to inject a lactated ringer/lidocaine injection solution into the subcutaneous fat. Following this, a liposuction cannula is inserted into a 60-cc syringe which is locked in the suction position. With a gentle rocking motion to and fro through the infiltrated lower abdomen, 20 to 30 cc of fat is obtained. A 60-cc transferring adapter adds additional saline solution to the syringe, and with a rocking motion the fat is cleansed with saline. The bloody saline is discarded and the process is repeated until the saline is clear. This provides golden brown fat. The syringe is placed upright and the fat is allowed to settle. The excess saline is discarded and the fat is then transferred to a Luer-lock syringe for periurethral injection through an 18-gauge needle. The second phase of autologous fat injection is similar to the injection of collagen in both needle placement and depth of needle placement.

POSTOPERATIVE CARE

Perioperative antibiotic coverage is continued for 3 days following the procedure. Most patients are able to void easily after the procedure, however if retention does develop clean intermittent catheterization is begun with a 12- or 14-French catheter. Indwelling catheters are to avoided in patients undergoing collagen and fat injection as this promotes molding of the material around the catheter. Although usually unnecessary, if long-term catheterization is needed suprapubic cystotomy should be performed in these patients.

Patients are contacted 2 weeks postprocedure in order to determine their continence status. Repeat injections are scheduled 1 month later as necessary.

RESULTS

Many studies have been extensively reviewed for efficacy and safety of PTFE by the Department of Technology Assessment of the American Medical Association[27] where it was concluded that it is a reasonably effective treatment for incontinence and technically easy to perform but, due to migration of particles and granuloma formation, the safety of the product remains uncertain despite the fact that there have been no reports of untoward sequelae in human beings. A study is currently underway comparing PTFE with collagen for both safety and efficacy.

The first clinical trial of collagen in humans for urinary incontinence was performed by Shortliffe et al. in 1989.[28] Sixteen males and one female underwent injection. Nine of 17 noted cure or improved symptoms and no granuloma or distant migration of the collagen material was noted in two patients who died of causes unrelated to the collagen injection. In the multicenter North American Study group[7] 306 patients evaluated by urodynamic testing underwent collagen implantation. In 137 female patients with ISD, 96.4% were reportedly dry at 1 year follow-up. In 17 patients with hypermobility of the sphincteric complex, 82.3% were improved or dry. Of the 134 patients with postprostatectomy incontinence, 78.7% were dry or improved at 1 year of follow-up. Admittedly, only 22 men (16.5%) were in the dry category.[2] Females with ISD required approximately 2.5 injections with an average of 24.3 ml of collagen whereas men with ISD required 3.9 injections with an average of 51.3 ml of collagen. Stricker and Haylen[29] noted an 82% success rate of the injection of collagen in the first 50 Australian patients to receive this therapy. While the success and efficacy of collagen implantation for females with ISD has been reproduced in several series, debate exists about the efficacy of collagen material in patients with Type II or anatomic stress urinary incontinence. A recent study by Herschorn et al.[3] reported equal success rates among patients with Type II or anatomic stress incontinence and patients with ISD, however the number of injections and the amount of material injected were higher in patients with anatomic urinary incontinence. It has also been documented that elderly female patients with anatomic incontinence do well with the injections of collagen material.[30] However, in our experience patients with hypermobility have not fared so well; in fact all 17 hypermobile patients in the multicenter study ultimately required surgical repair. In our hands the overall results with periurethral injections of collagen in females with ISD compare favorably with results obtained using slings and the artificial sphincter.[31]

With respect to the application of autologous fat injection for urinary incontinence, the male patients with postprostatectomy demonstrate poor results as well as women with hypermobility of the sphincteric complex. The 12 patients with ISD 83% were improved subjectively; however, this improvement rate appeared to drop precipitously at 1 year.[32] Therefore, although autologous fat injections seem to work reasonable well for ISD, the long-term follow-up needs to be assessed, as it appears that autologous fat undergoes a rapid rate of reabsorption due to its high water content.

COMPLICATIONS

Perioperative complications associated with periurethral injections are uncommon. The rate of urinary retention in patients undergoing PTFE injections is approximately 20% to 25%.[12] In the multicenter U.S. clinical trial of Contigen injections, transient retention developed in approximately 15% of patients.[7] Irritative voiding symptoms develop in approximately 20% of patients following the injection of PTFE, but resolve after several days.[33] With the Contigen, only 1% of patients experienced irritative voiding symptoms and 5% developed a urinary tract infection.[7] Patients following PTFE injections have noted the development of fever with negative blood cultures and urine cultures at a rate of 25%. This usually resolves after several days and probably indicates a mild allergic response.[12] Hypersensitivity responses with Contigen are not a problem, as the possibility is assessed by skin testing (wheal and flare) with the more immunogenic and sensitizing noncrosslinked collagen prior to treatment.[34,35] Those with a positive skin test are excluded from treatment and this amounted to 11 of 427 total patients in the multicenter U.S. study who, additionally, had anticollagen antibody testing and no significant anticollagen responses were found. There has been no evidence to link injections of bovine collagen with any disorder.[31] Regardless of the material, the use of periurethral injections has proven to be safe, eliciting only minor complications. All complications are rapid to resolve, and a serious long-term complication from the use of periurethral injections has yet to be reported.

SUMMARY

In our properly selected patients, periurethral injections offer excellent treatment results for patients with ISD. Patients with no anatomic hypermobility and ISD appear to be the most satisfactory candidates for periurethral injections. Contigen is the most widely used injectable, as it has been shown to be both biocompatible and biodegradable. There are no reports of particle migration with this material, and repeat injections can be performed safely under local anesthesia. Autologous fat is an alternative in periurethral injectable particularly in patients who have had positive skin tests to the collagen material.

In our opinion the treatment response in females with these procedures is similar to surgical procedures to correct ISD and the complications are minimal.[4] Of the alternative treatments available for females with ISD, sling surgery is successful in 81–98%,[36] implantation of the artificial urinary sphincter (either by abdominal or transvaginal approach) in over 90%,[37] and injection therapy between 64% and 95% of patients.[1] Although long-term results (>5 years) for all of these procedures are scarce in the literature, injected patients have been followed for only short periods of time and the data available does not take into consideration reinjection rates. In our experience, only 22% of patients who were dry for two years required a subsequent injection.[38] However, in males the success rate of intraurethral injections does not approach that of the artificial urinary sphincter to date. In selected elderly and less mobile female patients with anatomic incontinence, recent data suggests that collagen may be useful in this patient population. The use of periurethral injections in the treatment of ISD certainly has a role in the treatment in the properly selected patient, and allows treatment of incontinence in patients who are poor surgical candidates and may be denied other forms of therapy.

REFERENCES

1. Appell RA: Injectables for urethral incompetence. *World J Urol* 8:208, 1990.

2. McGuire EJ, Appell RA: Transurethral collagen injection for urinary incontinence. *Urology* 43:413, 1994.

3. Herschorn S, Radomski SB, Steele DJ: Early experience with intraurethral collagen injections for urinary incontinence. *J Urol* 148:1797, 1992.

4. Chrystle CD, Charme LS, Copeland WE: Q-tip test for stress urinary incontinence. *Obstet Gynecol* 38:313, 1971.

5. Appell RA: Valsalva leak point pressure (LPP) versus urethral pressure profile (UPP) in the evaluation of intrinsic sphincteric deficiency (ISD). Presented at the American Urogynecology Society annual meeting, Toronto, Canada, 1994.

6. Appell RA: Periurethral collagen injection for female incontinence. *Problems Urol* 5:134, 1990.

7. Bard CR: PMAA submission to U.S. Food and Drug Administration for IDE #G850010, 1990.

8. Sachse H: Treatment of urinary incontinence with sclerosing solutions, indications, results and complications. *Urol Int* 15:255, 1963.

9. Appell RA: The periurethral injection of autologous blood. Presented at the American Urogynecology Society annual meeting, Toronto, Canada, 1994.

10. Santarosa R, Blaivas J: Building continence with periurethal fat injections. *Contemp Urol* 5:96,
    1993.

11. Malizia AA Jr, Reiman JM, Myers RP, et al: Migration and granulomatous reaction after peri-
    urethral injection of polytef (Teflon). *JAMA* 251:3277, 1984.

12. Politano V: Periurethral polytetrafluorethylene injection for urinary incontinence. *J Urol*
    127:439, 1982.

13. Stegman S, Chu S, Bensch K, et al: A light and electron microscopic evaluation of Zyderm col-
    lagen and Zyplast implants in aging human facial skin: a pilot study. *Arch Dermatol* 123:1644,
    1987.

14. Remacle M, Marbaix E: Collagen implants in the human larynx: pathologic dissemination of
    two cases. *Arch Otolaryngol* 245:203, 1988.

15. Henly DR, Barrett DM, Weiland TL, et al: Particulate silicone for use in periurethral injections:
    local tissue effects and search for migration. *J Urol* 153:2039, 1995.

16. Press S, Badlani G: Injection therapy for urinary incontinence. In *AUA Update Series* 14(Les-
    son 2):14, 1995.

17. Appell RA: Collagen injection therapy for urinary incontinence. *Urol Clin North Am* 21:177,
    1994.

18. O'Connell HE, McGuire EJ: Transurethral collagen therapy in women. *J Urol* 154:1463, 1995.

19. Kegeyama S, Kawabe K, Susuki K, et al: Collagen implantation for post prostatectomy incon-
    tinence: early experience with a transrectal ultrasonographically guided method. *J Urol*
    152:1473, 1994.

20. Neal Jr D, Lahaye M, Lowe D: Improved needle placement technique in periurethral collagen
    injection. *Urology* 45:865, 1995.

21. Klutke C: Personal communication, 1995.

22. Pintauro W: Personal communication, 1995.

23. Winters JC, Appell RA: Antegrade collagen injections in males. *Urology* (in press).

24. Stanisic TH, Jennings CE, Miller JI, et al: Polytetrafluoroethylene injection for post prostatec-
    tomy incontinence: experience with 20 patients during three years. *J Urol* 146:1575, 1991.

25. Cervigni M, Panei M: Periurethral autologous fat injection for Type III stress urinary inconti-
    nence. *J Urol* (Part 2) 149:403A, 1993.

26. Ganibathi K, Leach GE: Periurethral injection techniques. *Atlas Urol Clin North Am* 2:101,
    1994.

27. Cole HM (ed): Diagnostic and therapeutic technology assessment (DATTA). *JAMA* 269:2975,
    1993.

28. Shortliffe LMD, Freiha FS, Kessler R, et al: Treatment of urinary incontinence by the peri-
    urethral implantation of glutaraldehyde cross-linked collegan. *J Urol* 141:538, 1989.

29. Stricker P, Haylen B: Injectable collagen for type 3 female stress incontinence: the first 50 Aus-
    tralian patients. *Med J Austr* 158:189, 1993.

30. Faerber GJ: Endoscopic collagen injection therapy for elderly women with Type I stress urinary
    incontinence. *J Urol* (Part 2) 155:527A, 1995.

31. Appell RA: Use of collagen injections for treatment of incontinence and reflux. *Adv Urol* 5:145,
    1992.

32. Santarosa RP, Blaivas JG: Periurethral injection of autologous fat for the treatment of sphinc-
    teric incontinence. *J Urol* 151:607, 1994.

33. Schulman CC, Simon J, Wespes E, et al: Endoscopic injection of Teflon for female urinary incontinence. *Eur Urol* 9:246, 1983.

34. Appell RA, McGuire EJ, De Ridder PA, et al: Summary of effectiveness and safety in the prospective, open, multicenter investigation of Contigen implant for incontinence due to intrinsic sphincteric deficiency in males. *J Urol* (Part 2) 153:271A, 1994.

35. Appell RA, McGuire EJ, De Ridder PA, et al: Summary of effectiveness and safety in the prospective, open, multicenter investigation of Contigen implant for incontinence due to intrinsic sphincteric deficiency in females. *J Urol* (Part 2) 153:418A, 1994.

36. Blaivas JG: Treatment of female incontinence secondary to damage or loss. *Urol Clin North Am* 18:355, 1991.

37. Appell RA: Artificial sphincter and periurethral injections. In Benson JT (ed): *Female Pelvic Floor Disorders.* New York, Norton, 1992, pp 257–268.

38. Appell RA: Collagen injections. *Urol Clin North Am* 22:673, 1995.

9

Neurogenic Bladder Dysfunction

Toyohiko Watanabe
David A. Rivas
Michael B. Chancellor

The empirical treatment of neurogenic voiding dysfunction, based solely on urinary symptoms, should be avoided because of the similarity of many of the voiding symptoms associated with various neurologic diseases. The interpretation of symptomatology alone is highly inaccurate as a means for the determination of the actual nature of detrusor or sphincteric dysfunction. Furthermore, symptoms secondary to neurologic disease are similar to symptoms that result from other common urologic conditions, such as pelvic floor relaxation and prolapse in women and benign prostatic hyperplasia and prostate cancer in men.[1,2]

This chapter will discuss the patterns of lower urinary tract dysfunction associated with neurologic disease, and enable the prediction of outcome and potential complications. New avenues of research, including intravesical drug instillation and neuromodulation for refractory neurogenic bladder dysfunction also will be discussed.

INITIAL ASSESSMENT

The initial urologic assessment should include a comprehensive medical history and physical examination. In women, the gynecologic and menstrual history is especially important in determining the extent of pelvic floor dysfunction. Pelvic examination may reveal vaginal atrophy, urethral hypermobility, and pelvic floor relaxation in women. In men, the examination of the genitalia and prostate are important to determine whether congenital malformation, malignancy, or an inflammatory condition may contribute to voiding dysfunction.[1,3] The urethral meatus should be closely inspected, especially in women with a chronic indwelling urethral catheter, as an eroded and patulous urethra may have developed.[4] Routine laboratory tests, including urine analysis, culture, and serum creatinine should be obtained. An elevated serum creatinine may herald significant upper tract deterioration in an otherwise asymptomatic patient. The evaluation of the upper urinary tracts is extremely important in patients with neurogenic vesical dysfunction, as hydronephrosis and vesicoureteral reflux may be responsible for compromised renal function. The presence of calculus disease, which occurs in over 30% of patients managed with an indwelling catheter,[5] may be evaluated with roentgenography or ultrasonography. Squamous metaplasia often develops from the chronic irritation of an indwelling foreign body, and squamous cell carcinoma can occur in up to 5% of patients.[6,7] Therefore, upper urinary tract imaging and lower tract endoscopy with mucosal biopsy should be considered part of routine urologic evaluation.

In the past, intravenous urography was most widely used as the preferred method of upper tract screening. Currently, however, ultrasonography is highly accurate as a screening tool for morphologic upper urinary tract changes and avoids the risks of nephrotoxicity and anaphylaxis associated with intravenous iodonated contrast administration. Nuclear medicine renal imaging is also effective for upper tract screening, although this method yields less anatomic detail but provides a greater objective assessment of glomerular filtration rate and differential renal function. Upper tract dilation may be further evaluated with a voiding cystourethrogram, to determine if vesicoureteral reflux is present.

URODYNAMIC EVALUATION

Urodynamic evaluation is the only means to establish the functional interrelationship of the components of the lower urinary tract. The purpose of urodynamic testing is not only to determine and classify a patient's type of voiding dysfunction, but also to identify risk factors such as detrusor–external sphincter dyssynergia (DESD) and decreased bladder compliance. Parameters of importance to be noted during a urodynamic evaluation include the capacity for urinary storage under low pressure, urethral closing function, and bladder and urethral micturition responses. Urodynamic evaluation describes a number of complementary tests of varying degrees of complexity that can be performed individually or in combination, depending on the clinical circumstance. Urodynamic tests vary from simple bedside "eyeball" cystometry to sophisticated multicomponent videourodynamic studies (Table 9.1). Some patients may require only a baseline screening study, such as residual urine volume measurement, while others receive benefit only after more extensive testing.

The selection of the most appropriate level of investigation depends upon the nature of a patient's problem and the availability of resources.[8–10] Advances in urodynamic equipment and technique have led to a significant improvement in understanding not only the normal function of the bladder and urethra, but also voiding dysfunction. Urodynamic evaluation has improved the ability to select therapy that addresses the underlying pathology of the lower urinary tract in patients with established or progressive upper urinary tract disease.[11]

It is imperative to reproduce a patient's voiding symptoms during the urodynamic investigation. If a woman with a neurologic disease complains of urinary incontinence, then to be useful, the urodynamic session should reproduce the incontinence in order to determine its cause.[12] In addition, it is important that the study be performed by a clinician who is experienced in urodynamic evaluation. The interpretation of a paper tracing of a urodynamic study, performed previously by a technician, should be avoided. The observation of

TABLE 9.1. Evaluation of Neurogenic Bladder Dysfunction

Neurologic evaluation of sacral nerves 2–4 reflex arc
   Rectal exam—Basal motor tone, sphincteric control
   Bulbocavernosus reflex
   Sensation of perianal dermatomes
Urine evaluation
   Microscopic analysis
   Chemical (dipstick) analysis
   Microbial culture and sensitivity determination
Incontinence evaluation
   Pad test
   Voiding diary
Upper urinary tract evaluation
   Ultrasonography
   Intravenous urography with tomography
   Computerized axial tomography
   Magnetic resonance imaging
   Radioisotope renal scan
   Retrograde urography
Cystourethroscopy (when indicated)
Urodynamic evaluation
   Postvoid residual urine volume
   Uroflowmetry
   Cystometrography
   Urethral pressure profilometry
   External urinary sphincter electromyography
   Video-urodynamics
   Multichannel studies
   Provocative testing:
      Bethanechol supersensitivity test (rarely indicated)
      Ice water infusion cystometrogram
Voiding cystourethrogram (if not performed as a component of videourodynamic evaluation)

the interaction of the detrusor, sphincter, and the patient's behavior is essential to establish the etiology for urinary symptomatology.

ELECTROMYOGRAPHY

Electromyography is an important component of urodynamic testing in patients with neurogenic vesical dysfunction. In the relaxed state, the normal urinary sphincter is generally electrically silent, with only infrequent action potentials. With progressive detrusor muscle contraction or bladder filling, a crescendo increase in external urethral sphincter electromyographic (EMG) activity develops, which reaches a maximum just prior to voiding.[13] Fibrillation potentials, positive sharp waves, and complex repetitive discharges may be noted in those with denervated muscle, but should not be present in normal individuals.[14] Increases in EMG activity usually accompany any cough, sneeze, straining, or movement.[15]

The beginning of a voluntary detrusor contraction is normally preceded by relaxation of the external urethral sphincter. At this point the sphincter EMG becomes electrically silent and the urethral pressure drops dramatically. Sphincter relaxation persists throughout the detrusor contraction, and at the termination of voiding, electromyographic activity resumes.[13]

Electromyography during urodynamic study is most easily performed using surface pad electrodes, rather than needle-type electrodes, because of the painless simplicity of application. Surface electrodes are placed on the skin overlying the muscle of the superficial anal sphincter and thus register potentials produced by the perineal musculature. Anal plug electrodes, utilizing two concentric rings mounted on an anal plug, may be used to more specifically measure superficial anal sphincter activity through the rectal mucosa. Similarly, two concentric rings can be mounted on a urethral catheter and direct measurement from the external urethral sphincter can be made. Although this type of EMG should be most accurate in theory, effective recording from sphincter electrodes is difficult to achieve in practice, therefore tracings often contain many artifacts.[16]

Although less comfortable, needle electrodes employing wire, monopolar, bipolar, or concentric electrodes are the most accurate method to record the EMG activity of the external sphincter.[13] The shape, amplitude, duration, and rate of firing of individual motor unit action potentials are observed on an oscilloscope during cystometry. When formal sphincter electromyography is not available, the simultaneous measurement of bladder and urethral pressure with fluoroscopic monitoring is useful in diagnosing detrusor-external sphincter dyssynergia in patients with spinal cord injury.

DIAGNOSIS OF URINARY INCONTINENCE

Type III stress urinary incontinence (SUI) results from a deficiency of sphincteric action, and is the type of stress incontinence most commonly seen in men and women with neurogenic lower urinary tract dysfunction.[17] This condition, where the sphincter has ceased to function, may result from denervation of the sphincter such as occurs with radical pelvic surgery or a cauda equina syndrome.[18,19] Alternatively, and more commonly seen among spinal cord injured females, traumatic sphincteric disruption may develop as a consequence of chronic urethral catheterization.[10] In such cases, ongoing catheter trauma to the bladder neck and urethra causes pressure necrosis to occur. In some patients with detrusor hyperreflexia, there is spontaneous expulsion of the catheter with its retaining balloon inflated, further damaging sphincteric function. In minor cases, the bladder neck and sphincter mechanism merely appear slightly open at rest, while in advanced cases irreparable injury results in a gaping defect.[4]

BLADDER DYSFUNCTION PATTERNS

Bladder and urethral function become altered in response to neurologic disease in a limited number of ways. This principle is critical to the evaluation and care of patients with urologic disability. Neurologic lesions produce either a loss of function, through a decrease in facilitatory nervous transmission, or a release of function, through a decrease in inhibitory impulses. Such loss of function is exemplified by paralysis of the detrusor in those with lower motor neuron lesions, whereas release of function is exemplified by detrusor overactivity in cases of suprasacral spinal cord injury.[20]

Patients with lumbosacral lesions, such as cauda equina injury and myelodysplasia, are more likely to develop a flaccid bladder. In such cases, facilitatory impulses are inadequate to generate detrusor contraction, therefore intravesical pressure does not develop and voiding does not occur. This detrusor areflexia, defined by the International Continence Society, is represented by the absence of spontaneous detrusor contraction in a patient with a neurologic lesion[11,13,21,22] (Fig. 9.1).

Alternatively, patients with suprasacral spinal cord lesions, such as those with traumatic spinal cord injury or multiple sclerosis, are prone to the development of detrusor hyperreflexia (DH) which may be accompanied with DESD.[23] Detrusor hyperreflexia denotes the development of detrusor contraction, during bladder filling, which occurs without the control of a patient with a neurologic lesion (Fig. 9.2).

In cases of DESD, inappropriate contraction of the striated urethral musculature accompanies involuntary detrusor contraction.[24] Since the detrusor muscle is contracting against a closed sphincter, dramatic increases in intravesical pressure develop. This high pressure can result in hydronephrosis and eventually cause vesicoureteral reflux. Urologic complications develop in at least 50% of patients within 5 years of the diagnosis of detrusor hyperreflexia associated with DESD[23-25] (Figs. 9.3 and 9.4) The incidence of urologic

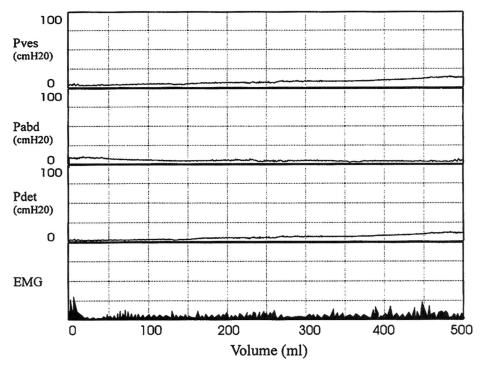

Fig. 9.1. Detrusor areflexia. A 34-year-old female 6 months after a motor vehicle accident resulted in crush injury to the pelvis suffers a cauda equina injury. Pves = intravesical pressure; Pabd = intra-abdominal pressure; Pdet = detrusor pressure (Pdet = Pves − Pabd), EMG = sphincter electromyography.

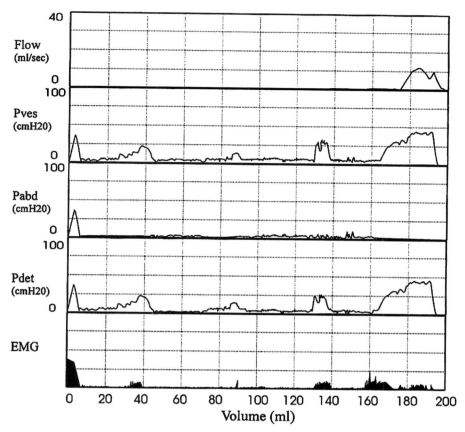

Fig. 9.2. Detrusor hyperreflexia. A 35-year-old woman with multiple sclerosis and urinary incontinence. During the urodynamic study, several involuntary detrusor contractions occurred. Flow = urinary flow rate; Pves = intravesical pressure; Pabd = intra-abdominal pressure; Pdet = subtracted detrusor pressure; EMG = sphincter electromyography.

complications with DESD is less in women than men. This is most likely because the lower sphincter outlet resistance of women does not permit pressure increases to the degree noted in men.

UROLOGIC MANAGEMENT

The ultimate goal of the urologic management of those patients afflicted with neurogenic vesical dysfunction is not only the preservation of renal function, but also the prevention of urologic complications. A discussion with the patient of long-term bladder management options is important in the early stages of rehabilitation. Of utmost importance is the avoidance of a chronic indwelling catheter and its associated complications of calculus formation, chronic urinary tract infection, neoplastic transformation, and soft tissue erosion.[5,7]

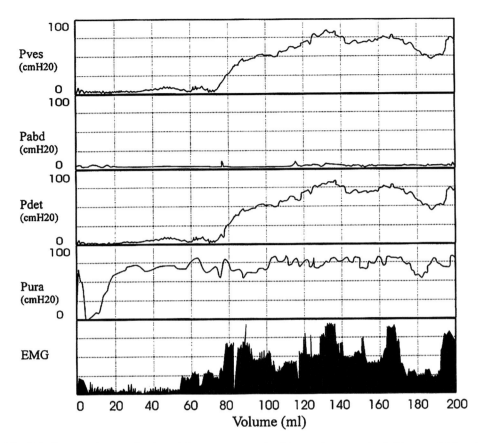

Fig. 9.3. Detrusor hyperreflexia and detrusor–external sphincter dyssynergia. A 58-year-old female with C5-level spinal cord injury voids spontaneously but suffers from urge incontinence. Detrusor hyperreflexia with DESD is exemplified by an uninhibited detrusor contraction occurring after 80 ml filling, a marked increase in EMG activity, and markedly elevated intravesical pressure. Pves = intravesical pressure; Pabd = intra-abdominal pressure; Pdet = subtracted detrusor pressure; Pura = urethral pressure, EMG.

Patient life style, occupation, physical home and working environment, and social factors must be considered in determining management selection.[26] The level of neurologic compromise may affect not only the degree to which lower urinary tract function is impaired, but also the potential for management options. An assessment of functional capabilities, such as manual dexterity and control of somatic muscle spasticity, should be taken into account. The availability of occupational assisting devices and attendant aid should also be considered[27] (Table 9.2).

Effective management strategies strive to achieve not only urinary continence, but also urinary storage and emptying under low intravesical pressure. Attempts at low-pressure urinary storage are usually made with the use of anticholinergic medications to suppress uninhibited detrusor contractions. If anticholinergic therapy is unsuccessful, surgical augmentation cystoplasty may be required to effectively decrease intravesical pressure to safe levels.[28,29]

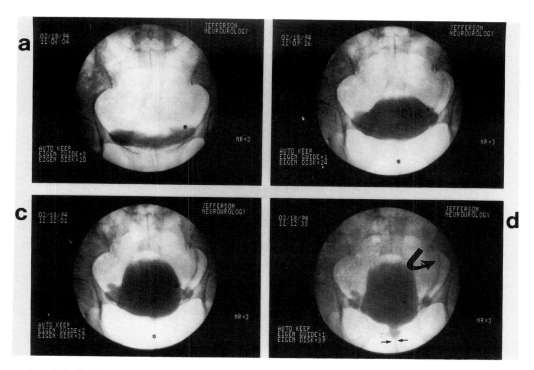

Fig. 9.4. Voiding cystourethrogram of a spinal cord injured woman with detrusor hyperreflexia and detrusor–external sphincter dyssynergia. **A:** The bladder appears relatively normal during early filling phase. **B:** Bladder near capacity. **C:** Initiation of voiding secondary to involuntary detrusor contraction. **D:** During voiding, the bladder neck is open but the urethra at the level of the external sphincter is significantly narrowed (*arrows*). Other findings on this study that are commonly seen with DESD are bladder diverticui and left vesicoureteral reflux (*curved arrows*).

TABLE 9.2. Patient Factors Influencing Therapy Option

Age
Desire to remain catheter- or appliance-free
Desire to avoid surgery
Economic resources
Educability of patient
Interest, reliability, and cooperation of family
Limiting factors including hand dexterity and ability to transfer
Mental status
Motivation
Prognosis of underlying disease
Sexual activity status
Rehabilitation progress

Decreasing outlet resistance will effectively decrease intravesical pressure. Employing external sphincterotomy to ensure sphincter relaxation is effective in men with upper motor neuron injuries, achieving efficient reflex emptying with condom catheter urinary drainage.[2] Decreasing outlet resistance in women is unacceptable, however, because gross urinary incontinence would ensue. Without an effective external collection device, significant perineal wetness results in significant complications. In women, therefore, urinary drainage must be accomplished with intermittent catheterization,[30] continuous drainage using either an indwelling catheter or urinary stoma, or spontaneous voluntary micturition, in order to achieve perineal dryness.[4]

SPONTANEOUS MICTURITION

Although it has been reported that some patients may be able to train their bladders and maintain continence, many have not found these methods successful.[17] The disadvantages of reflex voiding include not only the poor predictability of reflex detrusor contractions, but also their inefficiency at accomplishing complete bladder emptying. This results in elevated postvoid residual urine volumes.

In some cases, women with areflexic detrusors may void by increasing intra-abdominal pressure. The ultimate outcome may be satisfactory because of low urethral sphincter outlet resistance.[31] In practice, however, few women satisfactorily achieve bladder emptying with Valsalva maneuvers. Concern exists, moreover, that this method intermittently produces high intravesical pressure which could potentially damage the upper tracts.

Pharmacologic therapy plays a minimal role in improving detrusor contractions in those with areflexia or impaired contractility. Parasympathomimetic agents, such as bethanechol, do not appear to be efficacious in promoting effective bladder emptying in patients with neurogenic vesical dysfunction.[32] The smooth muscle–contracting properties of prostaglandins have been investigated through intravesical applications, although success has been limited.[33]

Sacral nerve stimulation, initially reported by Brindley, holds promise for future management options. In past investigations, neurostimulation results have been short-lived. Recent studies have shown that the sacral root stimulator can be satisfactorily used by those women with intact anterior S2–4 nerve roots to control voiding.[34] Long-term follow-up of these patients will hopefully reveal durable results.

DIAGNOSIS-SPECIFIC MANAGEMENT OPTIONS

Detrusor areflexia may be seen in patients with sacral and many lumbar level injuries. Management is generally sufficient with intermittent catheterization alone, although anticholinergics or bladder augmentation may be required if poor compliance results in excessive vesical urinary storage pressure.[35]

Detrusor hyperreflexia with synergistic external sphincter function may be seen in those with brain injury, incomplete, and nontraumatic spinal injury. Anticholinergic medications help control uninhibited detrusor contractions, thereby restoring continence.

Detrusor hyperreflexia associated with DESD is most commonly seen in patients with complete thoracic and cervical spinal cord injury.[36,37] While anticholinergics may control uninhibited detrusor contractions and thereby lower intravesical urinary storage pressure, intermittent catheterization is necessary to accomplish low-pressure urinary drainage. In those cases where anticholinergic therapy is unsuccessful in effectively treating a hyper-reflexic detrusor, augmentation cystoplasty may be required in order to achieve low-pressure storage.[38]

Alternatively, if outlet resistance is decreased, a decrease in intravesical pressure will occur.[39] Because men can utilize an external urinary drainage catheter, this may be accomplished with ablation of sphincteric function using sphincterotomy. In women, however, the resultant perineal incontinence is most undesirable. An alternative low-pressure urinary outlet may be established using an ileal conduit from the dome of the bladder to the anterior abdominal wall, a "bladder chimney." Over the long term, a cutaneous ileocystostomy is probably superior to an indwelling suprapubic tube cystostomy because of the elimination of the indwelling foreign body and its risks of calculus formation, chronic infection, neoplastic transformation, and tissue erosion.[40]

SPHINCTER ABLATION

It is best to defer considering surgical sphincteric destruction until it is certain not only that neural recovery after spinal cord injury is no longer progressing, but also that other types of nondestructive management have been unsuccessful or are not possible. Different surgical techniques have been used for external sphincterotomy, using electrocautery or a special urethrotome to incise one or more positions through the sphincter.

Anatomically, the bulk of the striated sphincter is anteromedial, while the neurovascular bundles are lateral to the membraneous urethra. Incisions at the 3 and 9 o'clock endoscopic positions are associated with injury to the neurovascular bundles of the corporal bodies and reduced potency. The 12 o'clock sphincterotomy, described by Madersbacher et al.[41] and Yalla et al.,[42] is the method of choice, because incision at this site decreases the risk of significant arterial hemorrhage and erectile dysfunction. Hemorrhage associated with the 12 o'clock incision usually emanates from venous structures, and abates spontaneously with catheter placement.

Complications of conventional external sphincterotomy include a reoperation rate of from 12% to 26%, hemorrhage requiring blood transfusion in 5% to 23%, and erectile dysfunction in from 2.8% to 64% of patients.[43–46] Perkash[43] has reported the development of secondary bladder neck obstruction in 26% of patients after external sphincterotomy. Therefore, any SCI patient with neurogenic bladder dysfunction must be followed indefinitely because of the risk of secondary deterioration. Several minimally invasive surgical alternatives to traditional sphincterotomy have been developed. Perhaps the two most promising for urologists are laser sphincterotomy and sphincter stent placement.

Laser Sphincterotomy

The performance of external sphincter ablation using the contact Nd:YAG (neodymium: yttrium aluminum garnet) laser permits carbonization as well as vaporization of tissue. Due to the near infrared wavelengths used, minimal laser energy produces approximately 4 mm of penetration per pass. Encouraging laser sphincterotomy results, with over 1 year of follow-up, have recently become available.[47]

The Sphincter Stent

The ingenious use of an endoluminal stent prosthesis to prevent sphincteric obstruction has been received with keen interest as an alternative treatment for DESD. Similar interest in intraurethral stenting has been applied for the treatment of benign prostatic hyperplasia and bulbous urethral stricture. Several intraurethral stents have been developed by private industry, however only the UroLume (American Medical Systems, Minnetonka, MN) has been systematically tested in the membranous urethra for the treatment of DESD.

The Multicenter North American Trial data of 153 patients treated with the sphincter stent has been recently published. Forty-four of the 153 patients (28.8%) had undergone at least one previous external sphincterotomy[48] A statistically significant decrease in voiding pressure and residual urine volume occurred in the patients with matched data from preinsertion values to postinsertion results at each follow-up period, up to 24 months. At 24 months follow-up there was no difference in all three urodynamic parameters between patients with and without prior external sphincterotomy. Neither stone formation nor urethral obstruction by endothelial hyperplasia occurred in this series, while subjective erectile function was not adversely altered in any patient. Ten patients underwent device explanation (6.5%), but of those, seven were reimplanted with another stent prosthesis.

The stent prosthesis continues to be an exciting, attractive alternative to external sphincterotomy. Besides demonstrating efficacy approximating external sphincter destruction, an improved safety profile, and decreased operative and hospitalization times, a major attribute of this device is that of potential reversibility. Spinal cord injury (SCI) patients tend to be eternally hopeful that medical science will someday develop a cure for their affliction. It is the permanently destructive nature of external sphincterotomy which makes the procedure objectionable to SCI patients. Conversely, the sphincter stent prosthesis is very positively accepted and requested by informed SCI individuals troubled with DESD.

CUTANEOUS ILEOCYSTOSTOMY

The establishment of low-pressure urinary drainage without the use of an indwelling urethral or suprapubic catheter may be accomplished by a cutaneous ileocystostomy, using a small section of terminal ileum to act as a conduit between the urinary bladder and the anterior abdominal wall; an ileal "bladder chimney." This procedure was reported in 1957 by Cordonnier,[49] but subsequently attention focused on augmentation cystoplasty and formal supravesical urinary diversion in treating those who might otherwise benefit from a bladder chimney.

The creation of a bladder chimney requires a major abdominal surgical endeavor, but is usually well tolerated by the patient. The patient is prepared for surgery with a full mechanical and antimicrobial bowel preparation. A 20-cm segment of distal ileum is isolated in standard fashion. The proximal end is spatulated widely and anastomosed to a similarly spatulated flap developed from the dome of the bladder. This wide anastomosis is required to avoid an hourglass deformity, which could impede egress of urine from the bladder. The distal end of the ileal segment is delivered to the anterior abdominal wall as the stoma of a Bricker ileal urinary conduit would be fashioned. The advantage of this procedure over standard cystectomy and ileal diversion is the avoidance of manipulation of the ureters, thereby eliminating the problems associated with ureterointestinal anastomoses such as reflux, stenosis, devascularization, urinary extravasation, or complete anastomotic disruption. Urinary collection is achieved with a standard urostomy drainage bag, without the need for an indwelling urethral or suprapubic catheter, which would predispose to chronic infection, tissue erosion, neoplasia, or calculus formation. Bladder capacity is preserved, and the gradual destruction of the bladder associated with indwelling catheters is obviated by this effective drainage procedure. Furthermore, the procedure is potentially reversible, as the bladder remains in place, with the ureters in normal anatomic position.[40]

The bladder chimney procedure has been undertaken in men and women with end-stage neurogenic vesical dysfunction and severe urinary incontinence after being chronically managed with indwelling urethral catheters (Figs. 9.5 and 9.6). In such patients, destruction of sphincteric function may mandate adjunctive therapy in order to ensure perineal dryness. In women, this is best achieved using pubovaginal sling urethral suspension to provide a functional urethral closure, rather than surgical bladder neck closure. Surgical bladder neck closure is reserved for the rare women where the entire urethra and bladder neck is destroyed.[50] In men with intrinsic sphincteric deficiency, the application of a gracilis muscle urethroplasty has been successful in achieving perineal dryness.

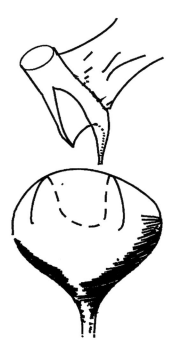

Fig. 9.5. Cutaneous ileocystostomy or "bladder chimney."

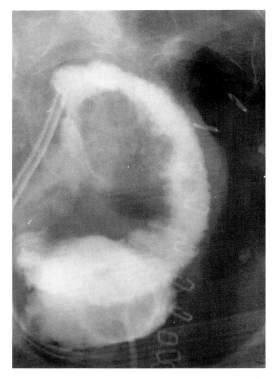

Fig. 9.6. A 27-year-old C5 spinal cord injured (SCI) woman managed with a chronically indwelling urethral catheter undergoes an ileocystostomy and pubovaginal sling procedure. Continence is established using pubovaginal sling at the bladder neck, while urinary drainage is accomplished through an ileal conduit from the dome of the bladder to the anterior abdominal wall (cutaneous ileocystostomy).

FUNCTIONAL URETHRAL CLOSURE

One of the most challenging problems in the management of women with neurogenic vesical dysfunction is the destroyed urethra secondary to chronic urethral catheterization. The resultant patulous, nonfunctional bladder neck and urethra has been termed intrinsic sphincter deficiency or Type III stress urinary incontinence.[51,52] A number of surgical operations have been described for its treatment, including the placement of an artificial urinary sphincter, cystectomy and urinary diversion, and surgical closure of the bladder neck and urethra. These procedures represent major surgical undertakings and risk the development of significant complications.[49,50,53–55]

Pubovaginal sling urethral suspension has been well described previously.[28,56,57] The sling is secured to the abdominal wall on one side and draped around the undersurface of the urethra at the junction of the bladder neck, then back to the abdominal wall on the contralateral side. The sling is fixed in position at its unsecured end with moderate traction on the suture.

The pubovaginal sling has been used for the treatment of stress urinary incontinence caused by intrinsic sphincter dysfunction, with therapeutic success ranging from 82% to

98%.[58] Complications of the procedure are primarily attributed to the excessive application of tension to the sling during its construction, potentially resulting in postoperative bladder outlet obstruction. In patients with a destroyed urethra, however, moderate tension is deliberately placed on the sling, thereby creating a functional bladder neck closure.

Suture closure of the bladder neck should be avoided because of the well-documented occurrence of postoperative fistula formation. In addition, in those patients undergoing a simultaneous bladder augmentation, a completely closed urinary system is avoided using pubovaginal sling urethral compression. This functional closure acts as a safety valve, enabling leakage, although at high pressure, to occur. This safety system avoids bladder overdistension which would result in rupture of an augmented bladder.[4,59,60] Although reconstruction of the bladder neck with a pubovaginal sling is performed for continence, leakage is anticipated if inappropriately high volumes or pressures develop.

THE CONTINENT CATHETERIZABLE ABDOMINAL STOMA

Despite the superiority of intermittent catheterization, up to 70% of women with physical disability are presently managed with indwelling catheters.[61] The most common reasons for relying on indwelling catheterization are related to a perception of increased ease of management, as the indwelling catheter requires exchange only once a month, rather than intermittent catheterization, which must be performed up to eight times daily.[26] In addition, catheterization in physically challenged females may be difficult, in that they neither can easily expose nor locate the urethral meatus in order to insert a catheter. One solution to this problem is the creation of a urinary stoma which is more easily accessed than the native urethra; a continent catheterizable stoma. This can be constructed concurrently during bladder augmentation or neobladder creation at the time of cystectomy. Concurrent cystectomy or creation of a wide vesico-vaginal fistula should be considered in most patients undergoing either incontinent or continent urinary diversion or neobladder. A fistula provides drainage of bladder contents, preventing pyocystis. It can be simply constructed by passing one blade of a GIA stapler into the bladder through the urethra and the other into the vagina. Thirty percent of these patients will ultimately require cystectomy because of the pyocystis which develops in a defunctionalized bladder, and delayed laparotomy to extirpate the bladder in such a patient with a major bowel reconfiguration is always difficult.

Bladder augmentation with a continent catheterizable stoma or continent urinary diversion in selected women is a reasonable alternative to an incontinent ileal conduit and certainly to indwelling catheterization. For those undergoing a neobladder procedure, the umbilical stoma provides an excellent cosmetic result which even patients with minimal dexterity catheterize easily. Such continent urinary diversion in women provides improved self-image and sexual experience.[62]

NEW PHARMACOLOGIC APPROACHES

Anticholinergic medications currently available are only partially effective in treating those with detrusor hyperreflexia. Significant undesirable side effects result in patient noncompliance. The development of newer agents, not only with the ability to eliminate uninhibited detrusor contractions, but also without bothersome anticholinergic side effects, is greatly in need. Currently available alternative options include medications with combined anticholinergic and calcium channel blocking properties, the intravesical instillation of anticholinergics agents, the analogue of antidiuretic hormone (desmopressin acetate [DDAVP]), and desensitization of bladder afferent input using intravesical capsaicin.

Terodiline Hydrocholoride

Terodiline hydrochloride, with both anticholinergic and calcium channel blocking activity, is a promising pharmacologic agent for the treatment of detrusor hyperreflexia. Tapp and associates treated 70 women with documented detrusor instability with terodiline and achieved encouraging results. The advantage of terodiline is efficacy similar to anticholinergic agents with less side effects.[63] It is unclear whether the anticholinergic or calcium channel blocking action of terodiline is primarily responsible for its clinical effect. After initially encouraging preliminary success, however, it is disappointing that terodiline is not available for clinical use. Terodiline has been voluntarily withdrawn worldwide, following reports of 36 cases of torsade de pointes ventricular fibrillation associated with use of the drug. Fourteen cases of bradyarrhythmia and eight deaths have also been reported.[64] The manufacturer is now reassessing this interesting drug, which may have applicability in the future.

Antidiuretic Hormone Analogue

Desmopressin (DDAVP) has been used for many years as an antidiuretic treatment in cases of central diabetes insipidus, and was introduced for treatment of nocturnal enuresis in the 1970s. A dosage of 10 μg can be conveniently administered as an intranasal spray at bedtime. DDAVP can effectively suppresses urine production for approximately 6–8 hr. Its clinical long-term safety has been established by continued use in children with nocturnal enuresis.[65]

Recently, DDAVP has been used in patients who have refractory nocturnal frequency and incontinence secondary to detrusor hyperreflexia. Kinn and Larsson[66] reported that micturition frequency decreased significantly in 13 patients with multiple sclerosis and urge incontinence treated with oral tablets or desmopressin, and that less urinary leakage occurred. Micturition frequency decreased from an average of 3.2 to 2.5 voidings during the 6 hr after drug intake. The manufacturer of DDAVP has not applied for FDA approval of this drug for use in adults with hyperactive detrusor function. DDAVP has helped decrease the frequency of self-catheterization and urinary incontinence in spinal cord injury patients managed with intermittent catheterization.[67]

Intravesical Treatment

The intravesical administration of medication has been used as an alternative to conventional oral ingestion for the unstable bladder. Intravesical instillation offers the potential for a high local concentration of drug at the detrusor muscle level while avoiding systemic side effects, because systemic drug levels are minimized. Several studies have reported the efficacy of intravesical instillation of anticholinergic agents for the treatment of detrusor hyperreflexia.[68,69] After their intravesical application low serum concentrations of both oxybutynin and terodiline have been detected.[70] It is unclear, however, if the low serum levels have a systemic, as opposed to a local, effect.

Appropriate candidates for intravesical anticholinergic therapy are patients with detrusor hyperreflexia who cannot tolerate oral anticholinergics. Our own experience with the intravesical instillation of anticholinergic agents has been only partially successful. The technique is cumbersome and requires that the patient learn self-catheterization. However, in properly motivated patients, or patients who cannot tolerate an oral anticholinergic regimen, intravesical instillation should be considered as a nonsurgical option.

Intravesical agents studied thus far include emepronium bromide, lidocaine, oxybutynin, terodiline, and verapamil.[71] Oxybutynin chloride has been the most studied of the intravesical agents. Oxybutynin tablets (5 mg) may be crushed and dissolved in 30 ml of sterile water. The solution is then instilled and retained intravesically for 30 mins 3 times daily.[72]

Capsaicin

Capsaicin, the pungent ingredient found in red peppers, is a neurotoxic compound that causes initial excitation, then desensitization, of unmyelinated C fibers of sensory neurons.[73,74] Capsaicin is capable of depleting sensory afferents of noxious neuropeptides, including substance P.[75] The potential clinical implications of being able to pharmacologically defunctionalize bladder sensory afferents is exciting.[76] Such an action would be ideal for the treatment of detrusor hyperreflexia and sensory urgency.[77] Intravesical capsaicin has been shown to inhibit detrusor hyperreflexia in a group of patients with multiple sclerosis.[78] The patients who responded enjoyed improvement for several months. No significant complications occurred in this series. Although potential problems exist with the mode of drug administration and undesirable sequelae of the initial excitatory effects, this is an interesting concept that holds promise for future avenues of drug treatment.[76,79,80] Encouraging preliminary results with the intravesical instillation of capsaicin have been achieved in neurologically impaired patients with detrusor hyperreflexia at our center.[81] Although intravesical capsaicin is an exciting and promising modality, premature embrace of this experimental concept must be tempered. The proper dosage, and frequency of administration, long-term side effects, and the impact of the alcohol vehicle used to bring capsaicin into solution must be carefully researched prior to its widespread use as a safe and effective therapy for neurogenic vesical dysfunction.[82] The safety and efficacy of capsaicin remains to be determined.

REFERENCES

1. Chancellor MB, Blaivas JG: Unstable bladder and anatomic defects. In Bushsbaum HJ, Schmidt JD (eds): *Gynecologic and Obstetric Urology*, ed 3. Philadelphia, WB Saunders, 1992, pp 371–400.

2. Chancellor MB, Rivas DA: The American Urological Association symptom index for women with voiding symptoms: lack of index specificity for benign prostate hyperplasia. *J Urol* 150:1706–1709, 1993.

3. Chancellor MB, Blaivas JG, Diagnostic evaluation of incontinence in patients with neurological disorders. *Compr Ther* 17:37–43, 1991.

4. Chancellor MB, Erhard MJ, Kiilholma PJ, et al: Functional urethral closure with pubovaginal sling for destroyed female urethra after long-term urethral catheterization. *Urology* 43:499–505, 1994.

5. Bunts RC: Management of urological complications in 1000 paraplegics. *J Urol* 79:733–741, 1958.

6. Bejany DE, Lockhart JL, Rhamy RK: Malignant vesical tumors following spinal cord injury. *J Urol* 138:1390–1392, 1987.

7. Bickel A, Culkin J, Wheeler JS: Bladder cancer in spinal cord injury patients. *J Urol* 146:1240–1242, 1991.

8. Hinman F Jr: Urodynamic testing: alternatives to electronics. *J Urol* 121:643–645, 1979.

9. Ouslander JG, Greengold B, Chen S: Complications of chronic indwelling urinary catheters among male nursing home patients: a prospective study. *J Urol* 138:1191–1195, 1987.

10. Wein AJ, Barrett DM: *Voiding Function and Dysfunction, A Logical and Practical Approach.* Chicago, Year Book Medical Publisher, 1988, pp 143–178.

11. McGuire EJ, Woodside JR, Borden TA, et al: Prognostic value of urodynamic testing in myelodysplastic patients. *J Urol* 126:205–209, 1981.

12. Sonda LP, Kogan BA, Koff SA, et al: Neurologic disease masquerading as genitourinary abnormality: the role of urodynamics in diagnosis. *J Urol* 129:1175–1178, 1983.

13. Blaivas JG: The neurophysiology of micturition: a clinical study of 550 patients. *J Urol* 127:958–963, 1982.

14. Siroky MB: Electromyography of the perineal striated muscles. In Krane RJ, Siroky MB (eds) *Clinical Neuro-Urology,* ed 2. Boston, Little, Brown, 1991, p 251.

15. Brown WF: The normal and abnormal spontaneous activity in muscle. In Brown WF (ed): *The Physiological and Technical Basis of Electromyography.* Boston, Butterworths, 1984, p 339.

16. Barrett DM: Disposable (infant) surface electrocardiogram electrodes in urodynamics: a simultaneous comparative study of electrodes. *J Urol* 124:663–664, 1980.

17. Lindan R, Liffler E, Bodner D: Urologic problems in the management of quadriplegic women. *Paraplegia* 25:381–385, 1987.

18. Smith A, Hosker G, Warrell D: The role of pudendal nerve damage in the aetiology of genuine stress incontinence in women. *Br J Obstet Gynecol* 96:29–32, 1989.

19. Snooks S, Swash M: Abnormalities of the innervation of the urethral striated sphincter musculature in incontinence. *Br J Urol* 56:401–405, 1984.

20. Kaplan SA, Chancellor MB, Blaivas JG: Bladder and sphincter behavior in patients with spinal cord lesions. *J Urol* 146:113–117, 1991.

21. Abrams PH, Blaivas JG, Stanton SL, et al: Standardization of lower urinary tract function. *Neurourol Urodynam* 7:403–405, 1988.

22. Blaivas JG, Fisher DM: Combined radiographic and urodynamic monitoring: advances in technique. *J Urol* 125:693–694, 1981.

23. Fam B, Yalla SV: Vesicourethral dysfunction in spinal cord injury and its management. *Semin Neurol* 8:150–155, 1988.

24. Blaivas JG, Barbalias GA: Detrusor-external sphincter dyssynergia in men with multiple sclerosis: an ominous urologic condition. *J Urol* 131:91–94, 1984.

25. Lloyd K: New trends in urologic management of spinal cord injured patients. *Central Nerv Syst Trauma* 3:1–15, 1986.

26. Jackson AB, DeVivo M: Urological long-term follow-up in women with spinal cord injuries. *Arch Phys Med Rehabil* 73:1029–1035, 1992.

27. Siosteen A, Lundqvist C, Blomstrand C, et al: Sexual ability, activity, attitudes and satisfaction as part of adjustment in spinal cord-injured subjects. *Paraplegia* 28:285–295, 1990.

28. Wan J, McGuire EJ: Augmentation cystoplasty and closure of the urethra for the destroyed lower urinary tract. *J Am Paraplegia Soc* 13:40–45, 1990.

29. Luangkhot R, Peng B, Blaivas JB: Ileocecocystoplasty for management of refractory neurogenic bladder. Surgical technique and urodynamic findings. *J Urol* 146:1340, 1991.

30. Lapides J, Diokno AC, Silber SJ, et al: Clean intermittent catheterization in the treatment of urinary tract disease. *J Urol* 107:458–461, 1972.

31. Merritt J, Lie M, Opitz J: Bladder retraining of paraplegic women. *Arch Phys Med Rehabil* 63:416–418, 1982.

32. Wein A: Pharmacologic treatment of lower urinary tract dysfunction in the female patient. *Urol Clin North Am* 12:259–270, 1985.

33. Delaere K, Thomas C, Moonen W, et al: The value of intravesical prostaglandin E2 and F2 in women with abnormalities of bladder emptying. *Br J Urol* 53:306–309, 1981.

34. Brindley G, Polkey C, Rushton D, et al: Sacral anterior root stimulators for bladder control in paraplegia: the first 50 cases. *J Neurol Neurosurg Psychiatry* 49:1104–1114, 1986.

35. Timoney A, Shaw P: Urological outcome in female patients with spinal cord injury: the effectiveness of intermittent catheterization. *Paraplegia* 28:556–563, 1990.

36. Chancellor MB, Erhard MJ, Rivas DA: Clinical effect of Alpha-1 antagonist terazosin on external and internal urinary sphincter. *J Amer Paraplegia Society* 16:207–214, 1993.

37. Chancellor MB, Rivas DA: Current management of detrusor sphincter dyssynergia. In McGuire EJ, (ed): *Advances in Urology*. Chicago, Mosby-Year Book, 1994.

38. Blaivas JG, Chancellor MB: Detrusor instability and incontinence: cystodistention, denervation of bladder, and augmentation cystoplasty. In Hurt JR (ed): *Urogynecologic Surgery*. Aspen Gaithersburg, Maryland, 1992, pp 102–128.

39. Rivas DA, Chancellor MB, Bagley DH: Prospective comparison of external sphincter prosthesis placement with external sphincterotomy in spinal cord injured men. *J Endourol* 8:89–93, 1994.

40. Rivas DA, Karasick S, Chancellor MB: Cutaneous ileocystostomy (bladder chimney) for the treatment of severe neurogenic vesical dysfunction. *Paraplegia* 33:530–535, 1995.

41. Madersbacher H, Scott FB: The twelve o'clock sphincterotomy: technique, indications, results. *Paraplegia* 13:261–267, 1976.

42. Yalla SV, Fam BA, Gabilondo FB, et al: Anteromedian external sphincterotomy: technique, rationale and complications. *J Urol* 117:489–493, 1977.

43. Perkash I: Modified approach to sphincterotomy in spinal cord injury patients: indications, technique, and results in 32 patients. *Paraplegia* 13:247, 1976.

44. Schellhammer PF, Hackler RH, Bunts RC: External sphincterotomy: an evaluation of 150 patients with neurogenic bladder. *J Urol* 110:199–202, 1973.

45. Whitmore WF, Fam BA, Yalla SV: Experience with anteromedian (12 o'clock) external urethral sphincterotomy in 100 male subjects with neuropathic bladders. *J Urol* 50:99, 1978.

46. Lockhart JL, Vorstman B, Weinstein D, et al: Sphincterotomy failure in neurogenic bladder disease. *J Urol* 135:86–89, 1986.

47. Rivas DA, Chancellor MB, Staas WE, et al: Contact Nd: YAG laser ablation of the external sphincter in spinal cord injured men with detrusor sphincter dyssynergia. *Urology (in press)*

48. Chancellor MB, Rivas DA, Ackman D, et al: Multicenter trial in North America of Urolume urinary sphincter prosthesis. *J Urol* 152:924–930, 1994.

49. Cordonnier JJ: Ileocystostomy for neurogenic bladder. *J Urol* 78:605–610, 1957.

50. Zimmern PE, Hadley HR, Leach GE, et al: Transvaginal closure of the bladder neck and placement of a suprapubic catheter for destroyed urethra after long-term indwelling catheterization. *J Urol* 134:554–557, 1985.

51. Blaivas JG, Olsson CA: Stress incontinence: classification and surgical approach. *J Urol* 139:727–731, 1988.

52. McGuire EJ, Savastano JA: Comparative urological outcome in women with spinal cord injury. *J Urol* 135:730–731, 1986.

53. Feneley RCL: The management of female incontinence by suprapubic catheterization, with or without urethral closure. *Br J Urol* 55:203–207, 1983.

54. Griffiths IH: Anterior transposition of the urethra. *Br J Urol* 32:27–31, 1960.

55. Mundy AR, Nurse DE, Dick JA, et al: Complex urinary undiversion. *Br J Urol* 58:640–643, 1986.

56. Blaivas JG, Chancellor MB: Complicated stress urinary incontinence. *Semin Urol* 7:103–116, 1989.

57. McGuire EJ, Bennett CJ, Konnak JA, et al: Experience with pubovaginal slings for urinary incontinence at the University of Michigan. *J Urol* 138:525–526, 1987.

58. Blaivas JG, Jacobs BZ: Pubovaginal fascial sling for the treatment of complicated stress urinary incontinence. *J Urol* 145:1214–1218, 1991.

59. Rosen MA, Light JK: Spontaneous bladder rupture following augmentation enterocystoplasty. *J Urol* 146:1232–1234, 1991.

60. Thompson ST, Kursh ED: Delayed spontaneous rupture on an ileocolonic neobladder. *J Urol* 148:1890–1891, 1992.

61. De Vivo MJ, Rutt RD, Black KJ, et al: Trends in spinal cord injury demographics and treatment outcomes between 1973 and 1986. *Arch Phys Med Rehabil* 73:424–430, 1992.

62. Moreno JG, Chancellor MC, Karasick S, et al: Improved quality of life and sexuality with continent urinary diversion in quadriplegic women with umbilical stoma. *Arch Phys Med Rehabil* (*in press*).

63. Tapp A, Fal M, Norgaard J, et al: Terodiline: a dose titrated, multicenter study of the treatment of idiopathic detrusor instability in women. *J Urol* 142:1027–1031, 1989.

64. Withdrawal of 'Micturin'. *Lancet* 338:752, 1991.

65. Rew DA, Rundle JSH: Assessment of the safety of regular DDAVP therapy in primary nocturnal enuresis. *Br J Urol* 63:352–353, 1989.

66. Kinn AC, Larsson PO: Desmopressin: a new principle for symptomatic treatment of urgency and incontinence in patients with multiple sclerosis. *Scand J Urol Nephrol* 24:109–112, 1990.

67. Chancellor MB, Rivas DA: DDAVP in the urological management of the difficult neurogenic bladder in spinal cord injury: preliminary report. *J Am Paraplegia Soc* 17:117 1994.

68. Brendler CB, Radebaugh LC, Mohler JL: Topical oxybutynin chloride for relaxation of dysfunctional bladders. *J Urol* 141:1350–1352, 1989.

69. O'Flynn KJ, Thomas DG: Intravesical instillation of oxybutynin hydrochloride for detrusor hyperreflexia. *Br J Urol* 72:566–570, 1993.

70. Jilg G, Madersbacher H: Intravesical application of oxybutynin hydrochloride for control of detrusor hyperreflexia. *Neurourol Urodyn* 8:312–315, 1989.

71. Ekstrom B, Andersson KE, Mattiasson A: Urodynamic effects of intravesical instillation of terodiline in healthy volunteers and in patients with detrusor hyperactivity. *J Urol* 148:1840–1844, 1993.

72. Madersbacher H, Jilg G: Control of detrusor hyperreflexia by intravesical instillation of oxybutynin hydrochloride. *Paraplegia* 29:84–90, 1991.

73. Barbanti G, Maggi CA, Beneforti P, et al: Relief of pain following intravesical capsaicin in patients with hypersensitive disorders of the lower urinary tract. *Br J Urol* 71:686–691, 1993.

74. Maggi CA, Meli A: The sensory efferent function of capsaicin-sensitive sensory neurons. *Gen Pharmacol* 19:1–43, 1988.

75. Maggi CA: Capsaicin and primary afferent neurons: from basic science to human therapy? *J Auton Nerv Syst* 33:1–14, 1991.

76. Maggi CA: Therapeutic potential of capsaicin like molecules: studies in animals and humans. *Life Sci* 51:1777–1781, 1992.

77. Sharkey KA, Williams RG, Schultzberg M, et al: Sensory substance P-innervation of the urinary bladder: possible site of action of capsaicin in causing urine retention in rats. *Neuroscience* 10:861–868, 1983.

78. Fowler CJ, Jewkes D, McDonald WI, et al: Intravesical capsaicin for neurogenic vesical dysfunction. *Lancet* 339:1239, 1992.

79. de Groat WC, Kawatani T, Hisamutsu T, et al: Mechanisms underlying the recovery of urinary bladder function following spinal cord injury. *J Autonom Nerv Syst* 30:S71–78, 1990.

80. Maggi CA, Barbanti G, Santicioli P, et al: Cystometric evidence that capsaicin-sensitive nerves modulate the afferent branch of micturition reflex in humans. *J Urol* 142:150–154, 1989.

81. Chancellor MB, Rivas DA, Byrne DE, et al: Intravesical capsaicin in neurologic impaired patients with detrusor hyperreflexia and autonomic dysreflexia: preliminary study. Research Symposium on Interstitial Cystitis. NIH, January 11, 1995.

82. Byrne DE, McCue P, Sedor J, et al: Acute effect of intravesical capsaicin on bladder mucin/glycosaminoglycan layer in control and spinal cord injured (SCI) rats. *J Urol* 153:262A, 1995.

10

Vesicovaginal Fistula

Ashok Chopra
Lynn Stothers
Shlomo Raz

Simply stated a vesicovaginal fistula represents a connection between the bladder and the vagina. Once an endemic problem related to obstetrical trauma, the etiologies and incidence have changed markedly in the last half of the twentieth century. Because of the proximity of the ureters and urethra, concurrent pathology in these areas may also be found. Techniques of repair vary and successful repair can be achieved through a variety of approaches. In this chapter we will discuss some of the management approaches available to the surgeon.

PATHOGENESIS AND ETIOLOGY

From a worldwide perspective, the leading cause of vesicovaginal fistula (VVF) is related to obstetrical trauma. Indeed this was the case in the U.S. until modern techniques of delivery and management became widespread. Currently, the predominant cause of VVF in the Western world is related to gynecologic procedures with about 82% of these injuries occurring in this setting (the abdominal hysterectomy is implicated in 44–74% of cases).[1,2] Other common causes include obstetrical trauma (8%), urologic trauma, radiation-induced necrosis of tissues (6%), trauma (4%), chronic irritation from foreign bodies, and carcinomas of the pelvis (primarily cervical, vaginal, endometrial).[2]

It is important to note that this chapter will address primarily vesicovaginal fistulas related to gynecologic trauma. Fistulas caused by obstetrical trauma and radiation have unique caveats of treatment.

DIAGNOSIS

The classic finding of VVF is a constant drainage of watery fluid from the vagina. Unfortunately the drainage may be quite minimal and the pattern of leakage difficult to ascertain. The history will often reveal a contributing factor such as recent pelvic surgery, a history of significant obstetrical trauma, or radiation. Chronological onset relates to the underlying etiology. Postsurgical fistulas classically present 1–3 weeks postoperatively (but may be seen earlier); fistulas caused by carcinoma or radiation may have delayed presentation of years.[3] Location of the fistula often relates to the preceding insult. Transvaginal hysterectomy is usually associated with trigonal fistulas; transabdominal hysterectomy is associated with fistulas at the level of the vaginal cuff.

If the volume of fluid is significant, this may be sent for creatinine level to determine its source. Alternatively, a variety of dye tests with the use of a vaginal tampon or packing have been described in the literature. One type of test involves placement of a tampon in the vagina with administration of pyridium. The tampon will be stained if the vaginal fluid is urine. A second technique involves instillation of methylene blue into the bladder. Once again the presence of dye on the tampon will confirm the diagnosis. In situations where the source of the fistula is unclear, a more sophisticated type of test may be used. In one such modification methylene blue is inserted into the bladder while the patient is using pyridium. A tampon is placed in the vagina. Pyridium staining of the tampon implies a ureteral fistula. Methylene blue staining of the tampon implies a vesicovaginal fistula (the presence of reflux may confound this test). A tampon that becomes stained with methylene blue only on voiding may represent a urethrovaginal fistula or reflux into the vagina.

A second method of diagnosis involves visualization of the vaginal wall while the bladder is filled with methylene blue or sterile milk (milk has the advantage of not staining the surrounding tissues). Direct visualization of draining dye will confirm the diagnosis; however, if this test is negative, the diagnosis is not excluded.

Radiologic tests include intravesical pyelogram (IVP) or retrograde pyelogram for evaluation of the upper tracts (approximately 12% of patients with vesicovaginal fistulas will also have ureterovaginal fistulas).[4] The bladder may be studied by cystogram (the single best radiographic test for vesicovaginal fistula diagnosis). When properly performed, the cystogram should include standing anterior–posterior films and lateral films with the bladder full. Care should be taken to consider vaginal or ureteral reflux as a confounding factor in evaluation. Urethral fistula may be demonstrated by this test or may be seen with a double balloon urethrogram.

Cystoscopy/vaginoscopy are diagnostic in most cases; however, the bladder/vagina may appear normal or may contain a patch of erythematous tissue but no distinct defect. Cystoscopy affords the opportunity for evaluation for a foreign body and also allows assessment of the size/position of the fistula and the ureteral orifices. The ureters may be evaluated through retrograde pyelograms, the bladder capacity assessed, and the urethra may also be examined. Finally, in the case of small uncomplicated fistulas, cystoscopy may allow for fulguration of the tract as described in the section on nonoperative and minimally invasive therapies.

TREATMENT

A number of caveats regarding treatment of VVF exist. It is vital that the surgeon study the patient thoroughly to uncover any injury to the ureters or urethra. The potential for multiple fistula in the bladder must be also considered. Viability of the tissues must be considered and an interposition flap may be advisable in certain cases. The bladder capacity may be decreased in patients secondary to radiation and/or chronic disuse. Patients with disuse atrophy generally will have gradual improvement of capacity after repair; patients with radiation injuries may, however, require augmentation at the time of fistula repair. If a suspicion of carcinoma exists biopsies must be taken, as the therapy will be altered radically in these cases. Concurrent pathology of the vaginal support such as urethral hypermobility, cystocele, vault prolapse, enterocele, or rectocele should be addressed at the time of surgical repair.

NONOPERATIVE AND MINIMALLY INVASIVE THERAPY

Nonoperative therapy has a limited role in the treatment of VVF. Small fistulas, however, on occasion, may respond to these therapies. Unfortunately, no major randomized studies exist addressing the success of nonoperative therapy. Available reports include that by Davits and Miranda in which they report on four spontaneous closures of posthysterectomy fistulas with 4–6 weeks of bladder drainage alone.[5] Falk and Orkin report on ten patients with vesicovaginal fistulas treated conservatively. Eight of these patients had fistulas less than 3 mm in size; two patients had fistulas that were larger. All eight patients with small fistulas responded to Bugbee electrocautery with 10 days of bladder drainage; the remaining two patients with larger fistulas failed this therapy.[6] Various authors have described treatment of small fistulas with mechanical denudation of the tract with screws or other mechanical devices. No good studies exist detailing response rates; however, it is generally advocated that these therapies be restricted to patients with small uncomplicated fistulas. Finally, reports exist on the use of lyophilized fibrin as a plug injected into the fistula.[7]

SURGICAL THERAPY

Broadly speaking, surgical options can be divided into transabdominal, transvesical, and transvaginal approaches. The use of various flaps may also be incorporated. In order to maximize the likelihood of success, various factors must be considered.

Timing of the Repair

Repair of obstetrical fistulas should be delayed in order to allow involution of changes of pregnancy and to allow traumatized tissues to heal. Further, because these injuries tend to be ischemic, delay allows for better demarcation of the extent of the injury.[8] Repair of radiation-induced fistulas should also be delayed (for at least 6 months) to allow tissue healing and demarcation of the extent of the injury.[8] One last group that requires delayed repair includes those patients with active infection in the pelvis (e.g., posthysterectomy cuff infections).

Gynecologic surgical injuries recognized intraoperatively should be repaired at the time they are recognized. Considerable debate exists over management of fistulas recognized postoperatively. The classic approach has been to delay surgery 3–6 months in order to allow tissues to heal. Certainly, in cases where a cuff infection is suspected (such as may be found posthysterectomy) a delay is always advisable.

Unfortunately, a prolonged waiting period can lead to considerable distress on behalf of the patient. As such, several authors have suggested the use of shorter waiting periods in select patient populations. The patient best suited for early repair is one with VVF status post transabdominal hysterectomy. In this situation repair may be performed transvaginally and is usually undertaken 2–3 weeks after the injury occurs. Raz reports success rates comparable to delayed repair for the transvaginal approach to uncomplicated fistulas.[9] Wang and Hadley have reported success with early surgical intervention for both high and low fistulas.[10] Blaivas compared early versus delayed repair and found no advantage to the latter.[11]

Desire to Maintain Sexual Function

Transvaginal repair of a large VVF may result in significant compromise of the size of the vagina. If preservation of sexual function is an issue, the surgeon may need to consider the use of flaps to maintain normal vaginal dimensions (or consider a transabdominal approach).

Hormonal Deficiency

Many patients who suffer from VVF will be hormonally deficient. Tissue integrity will be improved through the use of preoperative estrogen.

Excision of the Fistulous Tract

Several authors emphasize the need to excise or debride the edges of the fistulous tract prior to closure. For the following reasons we generally do not pursue this option: (1) Excision of the tract often incites bleeding which may compromise the repair. (2) Excision of the tract often changes a small fistula into a large fistula. In these cases a greater degree of tissue mobilization is required and ureteral reimplantation may be required. (3) Preservation of the fibrous ring at the edges of the fistula provides a strong anchor for placement of the sutures. Hadley and other authors have reported on layered closure of the defect without excision of the tract.[2,10] Outcomes with this technique (in this population) are comparable to those reported by authors who advocate excision of the tract.

Interposition of Tissue

A variety of flaps have been utilized in the repair of VVF. These include the Martius (fibrofatty labial) flap, the gracilis flap, various skin rotational flaps, peritoneal flaps, and omental flaps. All have the effect of improving vascularity to the tissues and providing an additional normal layer of tissue interposed between the two injured layers. Flaps are most often used in patients with radiated tissues, in patients who have failed previous repair, and in patients with large defects. Alternatively, several authors describe use of gastric or intestinal patches for fistula repairs. These techniques also interpose healthy tissue over the site of the defect.[12,13] Smaller defects in otherwise undamaged tissue may be quite adequately addressed without the use of such flaps.

Presence of Concurrent Pathology

As stated previously, a thorough assessment of associated injuries is imperative. Unrecognized ureterovaginal or urethral fistula can confound surgery. Additionally, care should be taken to address any pelvic prolapse (specifically urethral hypermobility and stress urinary incontinence).

In the remainder of this chapter we will discuss our technique of repair of VVF via the abdominal and transvaginal approach. The techniques of peritoneal, omental, and Martius flap development are briefly discussed here; the reader is referred to other sources for a complete discussion of flap procedures.

PRINCIPLES OF FISTULA REPAIR

Surgical principles in the repair of vesicovaginal fistulas mirror those for repair of other fistulas: (1) Tension-free anastomosis with use of flaps or relaxing incisions if necessary. (2) Use of well-vascularized tissue with interposition grafts if needed. (3) Resolution of infection. (4) Evaluation for carcinoma if clinical suspicion exists. (5) Multiple layers of closure with healthy tissues.

In the next sections we will discuss our technique of transvaginal repair and transabdominal repair. Transvesical approaches as well as interposition flaps will be briefly addressed.

Vaginal Approach (Raz Technique)

When possible we prefer to utilize the transvaginal route for repair of fistula. Raz, Wang, and Hadley have reported success with repair of both high and low fistulas through this approach.[2,10] The transvaginal route avoids cystotomy and allows for a shorter recuperation period. We reserve the transabdominal route for patients with coexistent intra-abdominal pathology, those with fixed and heavily damaged vaginal tissues, and for those patients who require bladder or ureteral reconstruction.

The Raz technique involved a six-step process for vaginal closure of a simple, uncomplicated vesicovaginal fistula. This repair results in a three-layer fistula closure. Other transvaginal techniques including the Latzko partial colpoclesis technique are not described; the reader is referred to the bibliography for further discussion.[14]

Step 1: The patient is placed in the lithotomy position following skin preparation with an iodine-based wash and vaginal douche. Cystoscopy and ureteral catheterization are carried out if the fistula tract is close to the ureteral orifices (single J stents may be left in place 4–5 days postoperatively in order to help keep the bladder dry). A suprapubic catheter is placed and left to drain. If the vault is narrow, a relaxing incision (posterolateral episiotomies) may be fashioned to aid in exposure. The labia are sutured apart and a ring retractor and weighted speculum are placed for further exposure.

Step 2: Saline is injected into the anterior vaginal wall surrounding the fistula tract. The fistula tract is dilated using metal sounds and a small catheter is inserted into the fistula tract which aids in retraction during dissection. An inverted J incision is made which circumscribes the fistula tract (Fig. 10.1). The long end of the J should extend to the apex of the vagina. The assymetric nature of the incision allows for later advancement and rotation of the posterior flap over the fistula repair. (For fistulas high in the vaginal cuff, the incision may be inverted with the base of the flap facing the urethral meatus.)

Step 3: Two flaps are dissected in an antero and postero direction on either side of the fistula tract. The ring of vaginal tissue at the fistula opening is left intact (Fig. 10.2). Creation of the flaps is begun in healthy tissue away from the fistula tract opening. This point of technique allows for dissection of proper tissue planes and avoids potential bladder perforation or expansion of the fistula tract. Each flap is dissected 2–4 cm from the fistula tract, exposing the perivesical fascia.

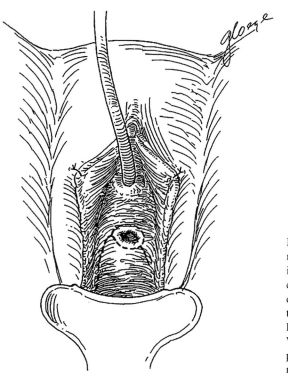

Fig. 10.1. The incision for vesicovaginal fistula repair is demonstrated. The incision is made to circumscribe the catheter placed into the fistula tract and extends in an inverted J shape toward the vaginal cuff. Figs. 10.1 to 10.4 from Raz S: *Atlas of Transvaginal Surgery.* WB Saunders, Philadelphia, 1992, pp 148, 150, 152. Reproduced with permission.

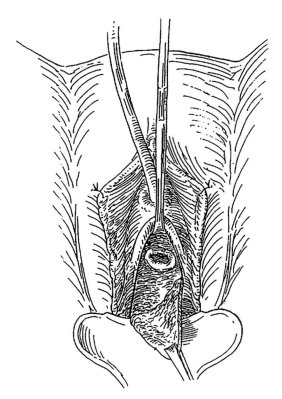

Fig. 10.2. Following the incision in the anterior vaginal wall, dissection is carried out in an anterior and posterior direction on either side of the fistula tract. The ring of the fistula is left intact. The vaginal flap should be generous in size and should be 2–4 cm mobilized from the fistula tract exposing the underlying perivesical fascia.

Step 4: The first layer of the repair is closed. The scarred edges of the fistula tract are closed with interrupted 2-0 absorbable sutures (Vicryl or Dexon) in a transverse fashion. A strong bite of tissue 2-3 mm away from the margin of the fistula is included in this layer which results in closure of the tract. These sutures incorporate the bladder wall and the fistula tract itself. After placement of these sutures, the intrafistula catheter is removed and the sutures are tied down. The second layer of the repair is then accomplished with interrupted absorbable sutures which are placed to invert the prior layer. These sutures include the perivesical fascia and deep musculature of the bladder. The sutures are applied at least 1 cm from the prior suture line; they should be free of tension and are placed in a line at 90° to the first incision line to minimize the overlapping components. The integrity of the repair is then tested by filling the bladder with indigo carmine (Fig. 10.3).

Step 5: The previously placed anterior vaginal wall flap is then resected. The posterior flap is rotated and extended beyond the closure of the fistula which covers the site with fresh vaginal tissue and avoids overlapping suture lines (Fig. 10.4). The vaginal wall should be advanced at least 3 cm beyond the fistula closure.

Step 6: A running, locking absorbable 2-0 suture (Dexon or Vicryl) is used to close the vaginal wall if no further adjuvant tissue interpositon is to be used. The vagina is packed with a triple sulfa-soaked gauze. A urethral Foley as well as the suprapubic catheter are left to straight drainage for 14 days.

Potential complications include bleeding and injury to the ureters. It is important to control bleeding and have perfect hemostasis. Hematoma formation may result in disruption

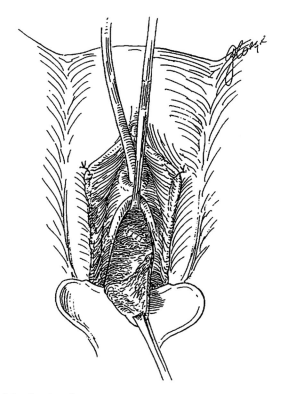

Fig. 10.3. Closure of the fistula prior to advancement of the flap.

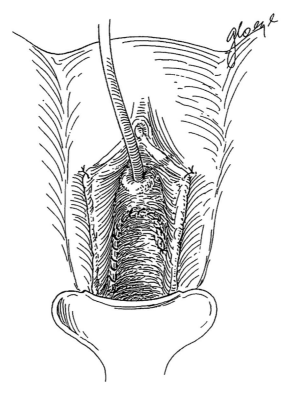

Fig. 10.4. Depiction of the J flap. The use of an inverted J-shaped incision with advancement over the first two layers of fistula closure avoids overlapping suture lines.

of the suture line and recurrent fistula formation. Bleeding encountered during the dissection of the vaginal flaps should be controlled with fine absorbable sutures and the use of cautery should be avoided. If there is doubt about injury to the ureters, the patient should be given 5 ml of indigo carmine and cystoscopy and/or ureteral catheterization should be carried out. The strength of the first two layers of closure is crucial to the success of the procedure.

Postoperative care includes placement of a vaginal pack which is generally removed within the first 24 h. Both catheters are left to drainage and are removed (in uncomplicated cases) at day 14 after the cystogram reveals resolution of the leak with adequate bladder emptying. Vital caveats for the postoperative care of these patients include continuous bladder drainage, control of infection, and control of bladder spasms. Vaginal trauma (e.g., sexual intercourse) should be avoided for 3 months postoperatively.

Delayed complications include vaginal shortening and stenosis, unrecognized ureteric injury or leak, and recurrence of the fistula. Recurrence of the fistula is the most common of these complications; repair may be done (either transvaginally or transabdominally) without delay. In these situations the use of an interposition graft is strongly recommended. Vaginal stenosis and shortening are associated with the repair of larger fistula defects. Ideally these complications should be anticipated preoperatively, however, if grafts were not performed at the time of initial surgery they may be performed after healing is complete. Initially unrecognized ureteric obstruction or leak should be treated with percutaneous nephrostomy to allow for a prolonged cooling-off period. Retrograde procedures such as retrograde pyelograms and ureteroscopy in the immediate postoperative period should be avoided as they may result in disruption of the repair.

Abdominal Approach

An abdominal approach to the repair of a vesicovaginal fistula is indicated when: (1) the abdomen requires opening for other concomitant procedures (such as associated augmentation cystoplasty for contracted postradiation bladders), (2) ureteral reconstruction is anticipated, (3) the vaginal tissues are heavily scarred or immobile, (4) the surgeon feels most comfortable with this technique. An abdominal approach is not always necessary when a previous vaginal approach has failed. Successful secondary vaginal procedures have been reported.[9]

Extravesical Approach

The extravesical transabdominal approach avoids the creation of a large iatrogenic cystotomy; the surgeon may proceed either intraperitoneally or extraperitoneally (more technically difficult). With this technique direct visualization of the ureters is not possible and adequate access to the defect may be difficult. Because of these limitations this technique is rarely indicated.

Transvesical Approach

Transvesical approaches to repair of fistulas may be categorized as intraperitoneal or extraperitoneal. Both procedures require creation of an iatrogenic cystotomy but allow direct visualization of the fistula and the ureteral orifices. In these approaches, patient positioning and preparation is identical to that for transabdominal repairs (frog leg with access to the vagina). Incision choices include the suprapubic "V", midline infraumbilical, or Pfannenstiel incision.[14]

Extraperitoneal transvesical repair of fistulas involves dissection of the bladder off the vagina at the level of the fistula via an extraperitoneal cystotomy. The repair is generally done in two layers with suture lines at right angles to each other. This technique provides difficult visualization and poor exposure; interposition grafts can not be used. As such, the intraperitoneal supravesical approach is preferred by most urologists.[14]

The *intraperitoneal transvesical approach* involves an initial incision with entrance into the peritoneum. The bladder dome is identified and opened. This cystotomy is used to visualize the ureters and the fistula. A catheter or stent is placed into the fistula defect in order to isolate this area (ureteral stents may also be placed if the ureters are in proximity to the fistula). The peritoneal reflection is taken down and the bladder is mobilized to the level of the fistula. At this point the cystotomy is extended to the level of the fistula using electrocautery (essentially partially bivalving the bladder) (Fig. 10.5A). The fistula defect (and any nonviable tissue) is now circumferentially excised (Fig. 10.5B). The vagina is repaired with absorbable suture; the bladder may be repaired primarily or with use of a bladder flap. If primary repair is undertaken, the suture lines of the vagina and bladder are oriented 90° to one another; if a bladder flap is used, the flap is rotated to cover the vaginal suture line. An omental or interposition graft may be used with this technique.[14] If the fistula repair encroaches on the ureteral orifices, they should be reimplanted; the fistula repair should not be compromised in an attempt to avoid this possibility.[14] A suprapubic

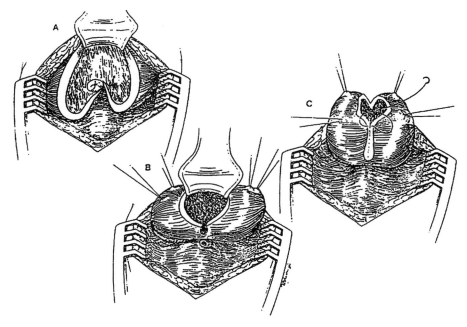

Fig. 10.5. **A:** Intraperitoneal transvesical approach. The bladder has been bivalved to the level of the fistula (no stents or isolating catheter depicted). **B:** Circumferential excision of the fistulous tract. The bladder and vagina have been dissected apart. **C:** Repair of the bladder with two layers of 2-0 vicryl. Suprapubic tube not depicted. Reproduced with permission from Gerber GS, Schoenberg HW. Female Urinary Tract Fistulas. *J Urol* 149(2):233, 1993.

tube is placed and the bladder closed with two layers of 2-0 Vicryl (Fig. 10.5C). A Jackson-Pratt drain is inserted. Postoperative care is identical to that for transabdominal repairs.

Results of Transabdominal Techniques of Repair

Many authors have reported on the success rates of the abdominal approach for vesicovaginal fistula repair. Success rates for primary closure range from 85% to 90% and are comparable to results for transvaginal repairs. Of note, these success rates are generally reported in those patient series without prior radiation; in patients with radiation-induced fistulae success rates tend to be in the 60% range.[9]

INTERPOSITION FLAPS

Multiple options exist for the creation of interposition flaps. Generally these can be divided into those best suited for the transvaginal approach and those suited to the transabdominal approach. A partial list of transvaginal procedures includes the Martius flap, the gracilis flap, the gluteal or labial flap, and the peritoneal flap. A partial list of flaps suited to the transabdominal approach includes the omental flap, the rectus flap, the peritoneal flap, and flaps made from appendix epiploica. Finally, it should be mentioned that bladder patches of bowel or stomach may be used to repair fistula defects.[12,13] Flaps are ideally suited for repair of complex, large or radiation-induced fistulas. They will improve blood flow to the site and also allow interposition of a layer of healthy tissue at the site of the defect. Rotational flaps may be specifically needed in those cases where insufficient vaginal wall tissue exists to complete the repair. The next section will briefly discuss the techniques of peritoneal flap, omental flap, and Martius flap. The reader is referred to the bibliography for a more detailed discussion of these and other techniques.

Omental Flaps

Use of the omentum is suited for transabdominal repair of fistula. In about 33% of cases the omentum will reach the pelvis without mobilization; in a further 33% of cases, division of the splenic vessels will be required to reach the pelvis; in the remainder of cases a more extensive mobilization will be required.[14] Generally, mobilization is based on a right gastroepiploic pedicle. This pedicle is used because of its usual dominance and its reliability. If further mobilization of the omentum is required, it can be performed by division of the omentum with strict attention to the vascular arcade.

Martius Flap

The Martius flap refers to a labial fatty tissue graft; it is well suited to transvaginal repairs. The graft receives its blood supply anteriorly from branches of the external pudendal artery, laterally from branches of the obturator artery, and posteriorly from branches of the internal pudendal artery. Either the anterior or posterior vascular supply can support the graft independently, allowing mobilization on either an anterior or posterior pedicle.[15] Harvesting begins with standard vaginal exposure and repair of the fistula. At this point, a vertical incision is made in the labia majora exposing the underlying fatty tissue. A pad of this fat is mobilized based on either its anterior or posterior pedicle. The lateral border of this dissection is the labiocrural fold, the medial border is the labia minora and the bulbocavernosus muscle, the posterior border is just superficial to Colles' fascia. This tissue is tunneled into position between the bladder and the vagina and is fixed in place with absorbable sutures. Hemostasis is vital and compression dressing to the labia should be provided postoperatively. Limitations include occasional inadequate length for treatment of high fistulas (especially in the patient with a deep vaginal vault) and atrophy of labial tissues which may be found in postmenopausal women.[16]

Peritoneal Flaps

The use of peritoneal flaps has been described in the literature as an alternative particularly well suited for the transvaginal repair of high lying fistulas.[2] It offers the advantage of simplicity and avoids the extravaginal incision required in a Martius flap.

In this technique the patient undergoes repair as described in the section on transvaginal fistula correction. After the first two suture layers are placed, dissection of the peritoneal flap begins in the anterior vaginal wall between the vaginal wall and the bladder. Dissection is limited to a superficial plane just underneath the wall of the vagina to avoid inadvertent cystotomy. The peritoneal reflection is exposed just beyond the posterior wall of the bladder in the anterior cul de sac. The peritoneal edge is mobilized (not entered) to cover the defect and secured with 2-0 polyglycolic acid sutures. At this point the anterior vaginal wall flap is advanced and the repair concluded. Raz reports on 11 patients who underwent repair of simple vesicovaginal fistulas with a peritoneal flap. In that series nine patients had complete response, one patient had recurrence of the fistula (which was later repaired successfully via the same technique), and one patient had rare leakage which resolved spontaneously after 6 months.[2] Since that report, 25 consecutive patients have been successfully treated with this technique (Raz S, unpublished data, UCLA, 1995).

Acknowledgment

The authors thank Ms. Connie Nelson for her kind and thoughtful support in the preparation of this chapter.

REFERENCES

1. Lee RA, Symmonds RE, Williams TJ: Current status of genitourinary fistula. *Obstet Gynecol* 72:313, 1988.

2. Raz S, Bregg JJ, Nitti VW, et al: Transvaginal repair of vesicovaginal fistula using a peritoneal flap. *J Urol* 150:56, 1993.

3. Kursh ED: Vesicovaginal fistula: post radiation therapy. In Resnick MI, Kursh ED (eds): *Current Therapy in Genitourinary Surgery,* ed 2. St Louis, BC Decker, 1992, pp 266–269.

4. Blandy JP, Badenoch DF, Fowler CG, et al: Early repair of iatrogenic injury to the ureter or bladder after gynecological surgery. *J Urol* 146:761, 1991.

5. Davits RJ, Miranda SI: Conservative management of vesicovaginal fistula by bladder drainage alone. *Br J Urol* 68:155, 1991.

6. Falk HL, Orkin LA. Nonsurgical closure of vesicovaginal fistulas. *Obstet Gynecol* 9:538, 1957.

7. Petterson S, Hedelin H, Tegee-Nilsson AC: Fibrin occlusion of a vesicovaginal fistula. *Lancet* 1:933, 1979.

8. Wein AJ, Malloy TR, Carpiniello VL, et al: Repair of vesicovaginal fistulas by a suprapubic transvesical approach. *Surg Gynecol Obstet* 150:57, 1980.

9. Zimmern PE, Hadley HR, Staskin DR, et al: Genitourinary fistulae: vaginal approaches for repair of vesicovaginal fistulae. *Urol Clin North Am* 12(2):361–367, 1985.

10. Wang Y, Hadley HR: Nondelayed transvaginal repair of high lying vesicovaginal fistula. *J Urol* 144(1):34, 1990.

11. Blaivas JG, Heritz DM, Romanzi LJ: Early versus late repair of vesicovaginal fistulas: vaginal and abdominal approaches. *J Urol* 153(4):1110, 1995.

12. Bissada SA, Bissada NK: Repair of active radiation induced vesicovaginal fistula using combined gastric and omental segments based on the gastroepiploic vessels. *J Urol* 147:1370, 1992.

13. Mraz JP, Sutory M: An alternative in surgical treatment of post irradiation vesicovaginal and rectovaginal fistulas: the seromuscular intestinal graft (patch). *J Urol* 151(2): 357, 1994.

14. Gerber GS, Schoenberg HW: Female urinary tract fistulas. *J Urol* 149(2): 229, 1993.

15. Elkins TE, Delancey JO, McGuire EJ: The use of modified Martius graft as an adjunctive technique in vesicovaginal and rectovaginal fistula repair. *Obstet Gynecol* 75(4): 727, 1990.

16. Raz S: *Atlas of Transvaginal Surgery.* Philadelphia, WB Saunders, 1992.

11

Products and Devices for Continence

Diane A. Smith

Ten years ago when embarking upon a career of conquering incontinence, this author only gave a cursory glance at absorptive products and devices. After all, most patients were going to be cured of their incontinence, and nurses knew all about incontinence products. As a specialist, very little advice was needed in this area. Right? *Wrong!* Many of the original patients needed much more help in choosing an appropriate product or device than anticipated. This chapter is intended to help both the novice and the expert in the basic and often overlooked area of products and devices for continence.

Appropriate assessment of the individual with urinary incontinence (UI) is essential before selecting and using continence devices. Patients need to be cured of urinary infection and fungal skin conditions, and treated to cure or reduce their incontinence.

No magical product can ever replace this treatment and cure. However, occasionally urinary incontinence is not cured or the patient cannot self-toilet and so creative alternative measures are needed.

LONG-TERM INDWELLING CATHETERS

Avoiding long-term use of indwelling catheters is the primary goal of any continence intervention. Use of an indwelling catheter should always be a short-term intervention used only for the comfort of the patient. In situations in which the patient has overflow incontinence or urinary retention and the client, family, or support staff cannot be available to perform or learn clean intermittent catheterization (CIC), an indwelling catheter might be the chosen option. Indwelling catheters can lead to sepsis, bacteriuria, urethral erosion, fistula formation, and an increased risk of bladder cancer. However, if an indwelling catheter is the best option, several points can be important in patient management. These include:

1. Choosing the *smallest* balloon and catheter size (16-Fr, 5-cc balloon). Obstruction is a consequence of many factors, but increasing catheter size only creates more irritation and leakage.

2. Encouraging normal bowel function and good fluid intake. Catheter irrigation should be avoided by ensuring good oral fluid intake. When bowel function is irregular, there may be urinary leakage around the catheter. Encouraging normal bowel function is essential in catheter management.

3. Several companies make coated catheters. These may be helpful in decreasing bacterial adherence but no clinical studies exist to prove this point. If the catheter is often obstructed, changing it every 2 weeks or less may improve the situation. Even the routine of changing the catheter every month is not substantiated by clinical data. Some papers suggest changing the system only when problems occur. Generally, this is not followed and a monthly catheter change is routine in nursing home settings.

4. Anchoring the catheter to abdomen or upper thigh is very important, especially for a urethral catheter. This helps to avoid erosion and irritation. Many companies make a variety of abdominal and leg straps. Insurance companies will often pay for these items. The urology office should have several samples on hand.

5. If the patient has an indwelling catheter and uses leg bags, teaching the patient to care for this equipment is essential. Generally, most nurses teach patients to rinse the leg bag and overnight bag with a weak vinegar solution. This solution is usually one (1) part white vinegar to three (3) parts water. Rinse bags with a catheter-tipped syringe and leave to dry.

There are a variety of leg bags from every company. Capacity and attachments to the leg vary significantly. A patient in the wheelchair may use an extension tube and a below-the-knee bag attachment. An ambulatory patient may not need an extension and may prefer a bag attached from the waist or a thigh bag. It is best to have a variety of products and to consider the daily life of the patient when making suggestions.

CLEAN INTERMITTENT CATHETERIZATION (CIC)

Teaching CIC is a skill learned through practice and observation. Often patients are unsuccessful in learning CIC because the staff is afraid or unfamiliar in teaching this skill. There are many teaching tools available for CIC. Mentor Corporation has videos available for patient teaching which show actual patients catheterizing themselves. These videos also address the emotional considerations of CIC. They can be obtained through company representatives.

Several companies (Bard, MMG) have catheter kits available for CIC. Many active patients prefer these kits, with a leg bag attached which makes doing CIC possible in the bed, car or train. After some experience catheterizing, most patients do this procedure by *feel* not *sight*. Teaching a patient to catheterize by feel from the beginning rather than by sight helps to avoid a patient feeling overwhelmed by learning the procedure. Balancing a mirror, light, and catheter is very difficult with only two hands.

Catheter extenders exist to make the catheter longer. A longer catheter facilitates catheterizing in the wheelchair and depositing the urine into a nearby toilet.

Special catheters for CIC are on the market and while most are made of rubber or silicone, metal and glass catheters are still available.

COLLECTION DEVICES

When the problem is facilitating toileting, collection devices may make a functionally disabled person continent again. There are many creative devices on the market. The most basic collection device is a toilet substitute, a device the client can use as a toilet when the toilet is either not available or unaccessible. For example, there are a variety of male and female urinals from which to choose. Often male patients who have hemiparesis can urinate into a regular male urinal but spill urine while removing the urinal. A spill-proof urinal with a flange that extends into the urinal and does not allow backflow even when held almost upside down is often called a rehabilitation urinal and can be very helpful. Sometimes, even a rehabilitation urinal handle needs modification and working with an occupational therapist can create a handle that is more functional so the patient can self-toilet. Of course, even the best urinal does not do a patient any service if it is not available or within reach. Additionally, time spent teaching patient to use the device is an important part of rehabilitation.

Female urinals are also an alternative for women on trips, in wheelchairs, or confined to bed. Female urinals are not easy to find in institutional settings, and often the device is only available through special medical suppliers. Key points to look for in a female urinal are ease of use and a flat side to facilitate use of the urinal in bed.

A basic funnel can also be modified as a female urinal. A large funnel with tubing attached can be used by the patient to urinate into from a wheelchair while the tubing allows the urine to flow into the toilet or commode chair. Many sports catalogs also have portable urinals which can be modified for this purpose.

The basic intervention of a bedpan is also worth mentioning. The use of a fracture pan makes the female patient more likely to be able to urinate without pain, especially in the period after a hip fracture or repair. Inflatable bedpans, like the Kimbro Pelvic Lift (Table 11.1), are also good alternatives for the patient who is in pain or difficult to turn and to move into position on a bedpan.

The Kimbro Lift is an inflatable bedpan which is placed under the patient like a draw sheet. It is inflated with a foot or hand pump and a pan is placed for deflation or urination. This device was created for the bed bound patient but can also be used in a wheelchair.

Newer collection devices are still being developed for functionally impaired patients. An example of this is the Dristar system (Table 11.1); this is battery-operated and mounted on a wheelchair or used at the bedside. This device combines a pad and suction to remove urine and store it in a compartment, which can later be emptied so that the patient remains "dry" at all times. Pads need to be changed two to three times a day. For a moderate to heavily incontinent patient, this device could avoid an indwelling cathether placement. Studies in the clinical use of this device are presently underway.

COMMODE CHAIRS AND TOILET ADAPTION

The simplest intervention for toileting is the commode chair. It is important to know that many different commodes exist, some with drop arms and adjustable heights to allow for tailoring the commode to the patient's needs. Other commodes are backless and can be placed over a toilet for quick adaption of a home bathroom. Changes in the bathroom can also enable a patient to remain continent. Removing the bathroom door and using a cur-

TABLE 11.1. Devices for Continence

Name of Device	Manufacturer
Kimbro Lift	Health Services Research and Development, Inc.
	10470 Waterfowl Terrace
	Columbia, MD 21044
	(410) 964-9678
Dristar System	EURO HEALTH
	3050 Redhill Avenue
	Costa Mesa, CA 92626
	1-800-Dristar
External Female	Hollister, Inc.
Collection Device	2000 Hollister Drive
	Libertyville, IL 60048
	(708) 680-1000
Female Urinal	Realmont Ltd.
	3300 2nd Street/Le Rue
	St. Hubert, Quebec, Canada
	(514) 443-2000
Pessaries	Milex Products, Inc.
	5915 Northwest Highway
	Chicago, IL 60631
	1-800-621-1278
Bladder neck	Johnson & Johnson Medical Inc.
support prosthesis	P.O. Box 90130
	Arlington, TX 76004-3130
	(817) 784-4984

tain or saloon doors can sometimes make wheelchair access possible. Placing grab bars at precise locations and using an adapter to raise the seat height can also make the toilet safer. Consulting a physical therapist, who is accustomed to modifying the environment to aid in functional rehabilitation, can be extremely helpful.

EXTERNAL DEVICES

External condom catheters for men have been used for many years. Over time manufacturers have made many modifications to improve the fit and reliability; however, not all makes can use a condom catheter. There are several factors to evaluate when considering this device.

The penile shaft must be of long enough length to support the device. If it is not, an external collecting pouch might be a reasonable substitute. Examine the skin on the shaft and if it is not healthy, consider using some protection, such as a barrier film, before placing the device. If the patient or caregiver must change the condom catheter, remember that a certain amount of dexterity is necessary, and the devices are not reliable for longer than 24 to 48 h. Usually changing can be accomplished during the patient's bath time. If the patient or caregiver must perform CIC with the device in place, placement requires more dexterity and care. However, Hollister, Inc., manufactures an external catheter which can be unscrewed at CIC time and then screwed back in place. This avoids placing a new condom catheter with every catheterization.

A strap to hold the external catheter in place is also helpful and manufactured by the Posey company. External catheters can be found with self-adhesives or applied with a form strap along the penile shaft. Self-adhesive catheters can be very helpful in patients with limited manual dexterity.

Some external catchers are made of latex. Latex-free products are important to know about when dealing with a disabled population. This is because "latex" allergy is a reported problem in patients who are continually exposed over time and so choosing a latex-free product may be important.

Do not recommend too large a leg bag; the collected urine will put too much weight on the condom catheter and gravity will pull it off the penis. Other suggestions are obvious but are often missed. These include starting with a clean, dry surface, shaving the hairs from the penile shaft, and using the heat of hand to help adherence of the adhesive in the self-adhesive condom catheters. The condom catheter must be applied smoothly. Do not allow a roll of the condom catheter because an ulceration may develop.

Because external female devices have not been overwhelmingly successful, several companies are developing urethral "plugs" or intraurethral "corks." None of these products are FDA-approved as yet although several are being investigated. These devices need careful research because they also carry risks due to their invasive nature.

PESSARIES

Pessaries are devices not to collect urine, but to support prolapse and provide urethral resistance in stress and mixed female incontinence. Some pessaries or bladder neck support devices claim to also correct urethrovesical angle and may be a nonsurgical treatment for female stress incontinence. This is helpful when surgical correction is unwanted or medically unsafe.

Recently a study by Davila and Ostermann showed a significant improvement both in reducing incontinence and in lengthening functional urethral length in a group of 32 women who were followed for 4 weeks of device use.[1] This device is called the Introl bladder neck support prosthesis and is manufactured by Johnson & Johnson Medical. The device was approved by the FDA in May 1995. This device is a silicone rubber vaginal prosthesis which is ring-shaped and has two blunt stumps located at one end. These stumps elevate the urethrovesical angle. This device is similar to a pessary in that it must be sized and cared for on a regular basis by either the patient or health care provider. Other incontinence pessaries and rings are also marketed by several companies. Besides those rings created for incontinence, any pessary may help support a prolapse or increase urethral resistance.

Fitting a pessary is an art simply because there are many different types and many sizes. Often the clinician can size and show efficiency of the pessary during a urodynamic evaluation. Demonstration that the use of this device reduces or eliminates UI can also be diagnostic in helping to decide whether a particular surgical procedure would be helpful.

Generally, pessaries should be removed, cleaned, and reinserted regularly. No studies report frequency of cleaning and removal.

If the device is made of silicone not rubber, it can usually remain in place 4–8 weeks. Porous rubber pessaries are usually changed daily by the patient or caregiver. The vaginal vault should be inspected regularly even if the patient is caring for the pessary herself. There is a reported increase in vaginal cancer with long-term pessary use.[2] For this reason, regular examinations and pap smears are needed.

Most clinicians who prescribe pessaries place patients who are postmenopausal on estrogen cream or oral estrogen. This practice is thought to provide a better mucosal lining in the vagina to support pessary use. A properly fitted pessary is not felt by the patient and does not result in abnormally increased residual urine. The patient should be told that occasionally a bowel movement (BM) may displace the pessary and she should be taught to "push" the device back into place after a BM. Pain or foul vaginal discharge should be reported to the office immediately. Bringing the patient back in 1 week to check pessary placement and to review teaching is a good practice after fitting and dispensing the device.

PENILE CLAMPS

Another device for males, which is not a collecting device, is the penile clamp. The external clamp prevents leakage by artificially closing the urethra. Several varieties exist. Clamps can be made of metal or plastic. Some are inflatable. When used inappropriately, clamps can cause ulceration and necrosis from the pressure on the penis. To prevent pressure problems, patients should never use the clamp at night, release the clamp if it feels uncomfortable, and release it every 2 hours to urinate. Generally, the penile clamp is most successful when used for short periods or during activities that usually cause UI, for example, while playing tennis or golf, dancing, or doing yard work. Fortunately, many men find the clamp uncomfortable and will abandon use of it on their own.

PADS AND CONTINENCE GARMENTS

The manufacture and sale of disposable and reusable pads and continence garments have become a multimillion dollar industry in the past several years.[3] Many people with UI turn to these products because they are easy to obtain and offer significant protection from accidents. Unfortunately, a dependence on such products can discourage patients from seeking help; they learn to live with the problem and manage it with costly products.

Disposable products have been greatly improved and offer more absorptive capability; however, they are costly to use and contribute to waste disposal problems. There are very few clinical studies which support use of one product over another. Currently patients choose a product based on availability, cost, and fit. This is, of course, an individual choice. Studies do not exist which describe skin condition, absorption, or durability of reusables. Clinical research is needed to correlate manufacture claims with actual use. Reusable products tend to be more expensive to purchase, but can save money in the long run.

Any continence garment on the body can increase the risk of skin breakdown because of the increase in skin temperature and the constant irritation of urine next to the skin. Meticulous skin care and frequent garment changes are necessary to prevent this. Barrier creams, ointments, and films can help prevent the constant contact between skin and wet garment and are less costly than any amount of wound healing.

When suggesting a product for a patient, consider the following guiding principles:

1. Be sure the product is necessary. "Just-in-case-protection" can contribute to UI, especially in the functionally or mentally disabled patient.

2. Determine the degree of protection necessary. Using a full garment when a small pad will suffice is wasteful and potentially damaging to the skin. Daytime protection needs may be different from the protection needed at night, so vary the pad or garment to match the need.

3. Match patients with products they can afford, manage, and obtain without difficulty. A great variety is available.

4. Keep several samples of pad and garment systems to show patients and families. Many patients rely on product displays in local grocery stores and are unaware of the great variety in cost, effectiveness, and fit.

CONCLUSIONS

Many devices exist to help manage or reduce incontinence. Not all of these products have clinical research data available to help make a scientific choice. Currently experience, exposure and an open mind are necessary to make the best choices for patients. Creative minds are needed to devise new products and to conduct much needed research.

REFERENCES

1. Davila CW, Ostermann V: The bladder neck support prosthesis: a nonsurgical approach to stress incontinence in adult women. *Am J Obstet Gynecol* 1994.

2. Schraub S, Sun X, Maingon P, et al: Cervical and vaginal cancer associated with pessary use. *Cancer* 69:2505–2509, 1992.

3. Agency for Health Care Policy and Research: *Clinical Practice Guideline. Urinary Incontinence in Adults.* Rockville, MD, Department of Health and Human Services, Report No AHCPR 92-0038, 1992.

ADDITIONAL RESOURCES

Hip Resource Guide. Hip Inc, Box 544, Union, SC 29379.

Ostomy Wound Management Journal, July 1995.

Verdell L (ed): *Resource Guide of Products and Services for Incontinence,* ed 6. Union, SC, HIP, 1994.

Index